THE ALLIED HEALTH PROFESSIONS

Also available in the
Sociology of Health Professions series

Support Workers and the Health Professions in International Perspective
The Invisible Providers of Health Care
Edited by **Mike Saks**

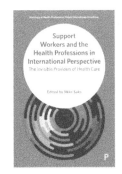

"...a well-written and informative discussion with analysis and description that has the potential to inform current and future workforce planning."
Ian Peate, Gibraltar Health Authority

HB £75.00 ISBN 9781447352105
242 pages July 2020

Professional Health Regulation in the Public Interest
International Perspectives
Edited by **John Martyn Chamberlain, Mike Dent** and **Mike Saks**

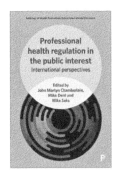

"With enormous variation in the delivery of healthcare, how it is regulated is more important than ever. The authors herein dissect the differences and enlighten us with forensic ability over a global range."
John Flood, Griffith University Law School

HB £75.00 ISBN 9781447332268
288 pages June 2018

For more information about the series visit

bristoluniversitypress.co.uk/sociology-of-health-professions

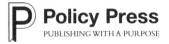

THE ALLIED HEALTH PROFESSIONS
A Sociological Perspective

Susan Nancarrow and Alan Borthwick

First published in Great Britain in 2021 by

Policy Press, an imprint of
Bristol University Press
University of Bristol
1–9 Old Park Hill
Bristol
BS2 8BB
UK
t: +44 (0)117 954 5940
e: bup-info@bristol.ac.uk

Details of international sales and distribution partners are available at
policy.bristoluniversitypress.co.uk

ISBN 978-1-4473-4536-7 hardcover
ISBN 978-1-4473-4537-4 ePub
ISBN 978-1-4473-4538-1 ePdf

Cover design: Qube Design
Front cover image: iStock/filo
Bristol University Press and Policy Press use environmentally
responsible print partners.
Printed and bound in Great Britain by CPI Group (UK) Ltd,
Croydon, CR0 4YY

Contents

List of abbreviations

ACT	Australian Capital Territory
ADL	activities of daily living
AHPA	Allied Health Professions Australia
AHPRA	Australian Health Practitioner Regulation Agency
AMA	Australian Medical Association
CCGs	clinical commissioning groups
CHM	Commission on Human Medicines
CWP	Changing Workforce Programme
DE	developmental educator
HCPC	Health and Care Professions Council
NHS	National Health Service
NRAS	(Australian) National Registration and Accreditation Scheme
ODP	operating department practitioners
OTA	occupational therapy assistant
PGDs	patient group directions
SCoR	Society and College of Radiographers

Acknowledgements

The authors would like to extend their heartfelt thanks to Mike Saks and Mike Dent, the series editors, for their advice, guidance and encouragement, as well as the opportunity to contribute to the series on the *Sociology of Health Professions: Future International Directions*, published by Policy Press.

There are a number of earlier works that have helped to inform and influence the present account of the allied health professions but two perhaps merit special mention. Gerald Larkin's marvellously articulate and insightful 1983 study of the allied health professions was a landmark text that retains its importance and vivacity to this day. So too does the beautifully crafted book on the sociology of professions by Keith Macdonald, published in 1995.

Mike Saks remains one of the world's leading academics in the field of the sociology of professions and, in our view, has contributed more to the development of the discipline than any other living scholar. For more than 30 years, his work has shed a keen sociological light on the health professions and has inspired a generation of academics in the discipline.

We are also indebted to Karl Heinz Schott and the Developmental Educators Australia Incorporated (DEAI) for their valuable contributions regarding the emerging professions of pedorthics and developmental educators.

Finally, we would like to express our genuine thanks to Laura Vickers-Rendall and the team at Policy Press.

Editors' overview

This edited text is the third in a series entitled the *Sociology of Health Professions: Future International Developments*, published by Policy Press and edited by Mike Saks and Mike Dent, supported by a high-profile international advisory board. The research-based series is focused on giving innovatory sociological insights into the past, present and future development of the health professions. It is mainly oriented towards final-year and postgraduate students, academic lecturers/researchers, practitioners and policy makers. Books included in the series must be resonant with the template for the general Policy Press series on the sociology of the health professions which aims:

- to inform and stimulate debate about issues in the sociology of health professions;
- to influence policy development and practice in the fields concerned;
- to make a significant contribution to academic thinking in the sociology of health; and
- to produce original national/international work of recognised high quality.

The importance of the current volume on *The Allied Health Professions: A Sociological Perspective* is in plugging a major contemporary hole in the literature in relation to the array of health professional groups that this book covers. The special significance of this monograph, written by Susan Nancarrow and Alan Borthwick, lies in the socio-political framework it provides in this area in the comparative context of Australia and the United Kingdom. The authors have unparalleled insight into the history and present operation of the often-neglected diverse range of health professions in these societies. In this light, we very much welcome this new addition to the Policy Press series on the sociology of the health professions – following books on *Professional Health Regulation in the Public Interest* and *Support Workers and the Health Professions in International Perspective*, with more commissioned work in process on subjects such as medical policy and dentistry on the international stage.

Mike Saks and Mike Dent

Introduction

This book helps to prepare allied health professions for a new and different future by telling the story of their past – specifically, the sociological, economic, political and philosophical pressures that have shaped the professions. For most of the past half-century, the allied health professions have focused on creating legitimacy through the pursuit of research evidence and the standardisation of practice. Yet, there has been very little analysis or understanding of who the allied health professions are – either individually or collectively – how and why they have developed, and their role and relationship to the health system and other professions. This book helps to address this gap in order to give the allied health professions the tools they need to navigate the sociopolitical landscape of the future.

Many allied health professions have ancient origins; however, the concept of the collective of 'allied health' as a group of professions is only decades old. Allied health professions can make an important contribution to society; however, in many cases, that contribution is not fully realised because allied health is poorly understood and largely underutilised. Many allied health professions have only recently professionalised, and new professions continue to emerge. At the same time, changing population demographics, new technologies and a shift in emphasis towards the management and prevention of chronic illness create a constantly changing landscape for the health workforce. This means that allied health professions are having to develop and shape their identity in a dynamic landscape.

This book compares the allied health professions, both as a collective and as individual disciplines, in Australia and the UK. Australia and the UK were chosen as a basis for comparison because the allied health professions have emerged in each jurisdiction from similar philosophies, regulatory structures and training approaches, which allows meaningful comparison. The different funding and system contexts provide a comparative basis to understand the impact of different features on allied health professionalisation.

We start from the position of the similarities between the allied health contexts in both countries. Politically, neo-liberalism has been influential in driving the healthcare funding models and accountabilities in both nations, though different healthcare funding systems have facilitated varied flexibilities within the allied health workforces in each context. The centralised model of the National Health Service (NHS) in the UK has explicitly driven workforce flexibilities and substitution between and within professions (both intra-allied health and between allied health, medicine and nursing). The more fragmented Australian funding system has created more obstacles for workforce flexibilities and, in some cases, limited options for professional expansion, which are otherwise available in the UK, but it does create the conditions for new professions to emerge. Despite these differences, the arguments for professional evolution have been similar, as have the contested areas of the workforce. The different contexts provide a valuable backdrop to compare the negotiation of the allied health professional project.

A textbook addressing the sociology of the allied health professions may attract several different audiences. It may offer insights into the allied health professions for those unfamiliar with them, and it may offer some theoretically informed explanations that help allied health professionals make greater sense of their world and place within the health division of labour. Sociologists may value a deeper understanding of what 'allied health professions' are, what they do, where they work and with whom, while allied health professionals may value the insights that theoretically informed, sociohistorical and contemporary sociological accounts can provide. Both, alongside other interested parties, may gain from accounts that explain in detail how the past continues to shape the present and inform the future.

Most allied health professionals have a firm sense of what and who they are, yet often seem puzzled that the public and other audiences do not share their perspectives. It is not uncommon for allied health professionals to express a need to educate, inform and enlighten others as to their roles, or to lament a seeming lack of understanding of their skills, contribution and place in the world of healthcare. By comparison, nursing and medicine are felt to be better understood, more appreciated and more clearly recognised for their skills. Yet, depending on the definition of allied health, they constitute at least a quarter of the healthcare workforce in the UK and in Australia (see: https://ahpa.com.au/allied-health/). Why, then, are they so ill understood? What are they and how did they become known as 'allied health' professions? In what way and to whom are they 'allied', and what role do they play in the broader division of healthcare?

Answering these questions requires an understanding of historical antecedents and context, as well as a broader appreciation of how professions emerge, develop and change. How should we view them?

Are they masters of their own destinies, shaping and transforming themselves at will, or merely matchsticks floating in the ocean, buffeted by waves and carried by currents beyond their control? Questions such as these demand careful analyses and coherent theoretical explanations. If we are to understand the 'allied' health professions, we must appreciate the broader health division of labour within which they work, how it is structured and how it operates. It is also necessary to appreciate and understand why occupations like these seek recognition as professions, as well as what they do to achieve and maintain it. Who do they need to convince in order to succeed? What are the external influences that shape or constrain the attainment of these goals? Sociological approaches, it will be argued, offer a window looking out over this landscape, providing the necessary insights that help to explain why these professions are 'allied', medically related but 'non-medical', and how they emerged from earlier phases in which they were 'allied to medicine', 'supplementary to medicine' and 'medical auxiliaries'.

The COVID-19 coronavirus pandemic dramatically and rapidly reshaped the way that healthcare is delivered in the 21st century (Smith et al, 2020). Significant and rapid innovations included: the removal or relaxation of practice restrictions for specific types of workers; an unprecedented uptake of e-health; the retraining and reskilling of allied health practitioners (and others) to take on shortage roles in areas such as intensive care and general medical wards; and the retraining and return to work of retired health workers. Services have been impacted as well. The intermittent cessation of elective surgery resulted in many patients being redirected to allied health services for the conservative management of conditions (such as the treatment of hip and knee arthritis). Some of these changes required rapid legislative changes to ease practice restrictions; others were enabled by the removal of bureaucratic restrictions (such as providing state funding for telehealth) (Bashshur et al, 2020; Smith et al, 2020).

Historically, allied health professions have responded well to crises. For example, the Second World War created substantial demand for rehabilitation-focused allied health practitioners, such as occupational therapists and physiotherapists. Shortages in medical personnel saw others, such as podiatrists, performing minor surgery, suturing and administering local anaesthetics. These skills were important in shaping the future skills repertoires of the professions. While the long-term impact of COVID-19 on society in general and the workforce in particular remains to be seen, the learning from the history and sociology of the professions contained in this book provides important tools to help allied health professions shape their future roles in the healthcare workforce.

The modern allied health professions were heavily shaped by the formal organisation of labour that emerged within the colonies of the British Empire as a result of the Industrial Revolution. This context is important for understanding the unique set of sociopolitical circumstances that shaped: their philosophies and scopes of practice; their interactions with other professions and society; and the diversity (or otherwise) of their workforces. Consequently, this book is largely focused on the way in which the allied health professions have emerged and developed within a Western context. Much of the sociological literature on the professions has been similarly focused given the difficulties in cross-national comparisons, which must take account of widely differing legal frameworks, regulation, sociopolitical structures and cultural variations (Collins, 1990a, 1990b; Torstendahl, 1990; Macdonald, 1995). Equally, there is a dearth of literature on allied health professions beyond the relatively narrow confines of the Western, anglophone world. Apart from the occasional insights captured in studies from Africa, Asia and the Middle East, available research is sparse (Awaad, 2003; Yang et al, 2006; Al Busaidy and Borthwick, 2012; Tawiah et al, 2018). To some extent, in the study of the more traditional professions (such as medicine or law), it is still possible to advance effective and meaningful cross-cultural comparisons, as is most evident in the work of Macdonald (1995) and especially that of Saks (2018); however, the paucity of data on the allied health professions restricts the scope of any comparable effort. The similar sociopolitical and cultural contexts important in the development of the allied health professions remains most evident in the case of Australia and the UK, and their emergent collective identity appears particularly unique to these nations. It is for that reason that the book focuses its attention on allied health in these two nations.

One key starting point is to examine and identify clearly who and what constitute the 'allied health professions'. The title 'allied' suggests a coherent and lasting bond between a core or close-knit group of healthcare professions that share certain features in common. However, most sociohistorical analyses of these professions point to a rather disparate group of professions located within a complex hierarchy of professional occupations in the healthcare division of labour (Larkin, 1983; Saks, 1983; Turner, 1995). Perhaps what they share is a social space or position within the healthcare hierarchy and a desire to enhance it. In this perspective, the profession of medicine sits atop the hierarchy, under which reside a number of less prestigious or powerful occupational groups, vying for recognition, legitimacy and status (Larkin, 1983; Saks, 1983, 1995, 2010, 2018; Freidson, 1988).

However, the allied health professions do not really comprise a clearly delineated group of health professions that are logically bound together by virtue of service ethic, skill range, purpose or boundaries. Nor is it immediately clear to whom they are allied; is it each other, or medicine, or perhaps something else? A glance at the current lists of 'allied health' professions, and by whom they are so classified, may give some pointers to the complexity involved. 'Allied health' professions are recognised as a formal grouping in both Australia and the UK but are not necessarily defined in this way elsewhere. Nor do the Australian and UK versions reflect the same group of professions. Definitions even vary within a single country. In the UK, for example, the Allied Health Professions Federation (AHPF), an organisation populated by and drawn from its constituent professional bodies, represents a group of 12 'allied' health professions, including podiatry, radiography, occupational therapy, orthoptics, prosthetists and orthotists, paramedics, physiotherapy, speech and language therapy, dramatherapy, art therapy, music therapy, and dietetics. It provides a common platform with which to lobby and inform government and other external agencies through one collective voice. However, NHS England currently recognises 14 'allied health' professions, additionally including operating department practitioners (ODPs) and osteopathy (see: www.england.nhs.uk/ahp/role/). Furthermore, the regulatory body, the Health and Care Professions Council (HCPC), registers 16 professions, adding hearing aid dispensers, clinical scientists and biomedical scientists, alongside practitioner psychologists and social workers, though these are not generally regarded as 'allied health' professions (see: www.hcpc-uk.org/about-us/who-we-regulate/the-professions/). Osteopathy, the most recent addition to the 'allied health' fold, was previously regarded as part of the 'complementary and alternative medicine' group of professions, and as such rather marginal to mainstream healthcare, lacking in the legitimacy afforded to more 'orthodox' professions (Saks, 1995; Turner, 1995).

In Australia, Allied Health Professions Australia (AHPA) – a national body representing the constituent professional groups that aims to provide a 'unified voice' to lobby and inform government and other key stakeholders, not unlike the AHPF in the UK – formally recognised 21 professions in 2020, including exercise physiology, chiropractic, audiology, genetic counselling, optometry, perfusion, rehabilitation counselling, social work, psychology and sonography, which are not recognised as 'allied health professions' in the UK.

However, it is worth pointing out that the AHPA is an independent group with no statutory authority (see: https://ahpa.com.au/allied-health-professions/). Curiously, the 'allied health professions' tend to be defined by what they are not, rather than what they are, particularly if viewed ahistorically. For example, the AHPA defines 'allied health' as a group of professions that are 'not medical, nursing or dental professions' (see: https://ahpa.com.au/what-is-allied-health/). Equally, the Department of Health allied health workforce review notes that the 'impetus to utilise the term and to be viewed as a "collective profession"' was related to the drive to enable greater autonomy while 'symbolising integration within the health system' (Mason, 2013: 300). To add to the confusion, each Australian state recognises a different suite of professions as allied health. For example, the state of Victoria acknowledges 27 professions as 'allied health', further divided into two branches – 'therapy' and 'science' (see: www2.health.vic.gov.au/health-workforce/allied-health-workforce/allied-health-professions) – whereas Queensland recognised 23 different professions in 2020, many of which are not recognised by the AHPA.

How can we conceptualise 'allied health' in the face of such difficulties? It may be more revealing and meaningful to examine the sociohistorical context through which the allied health professions came to be grouped together, why they emerged as a collective and how the constituent occupational groups have changed over time. Examining the processes of professionalisation at work in shaping these changes, underpinned by social theory based on empirically sound exemplars, perhaps offers the best hope of understanding what has happened in the past, what is going on now and where it may be leading the allied health professions in future.

The allied health professions

It is abundantly clear that in many Western nations, the healthcare division of labour includes a range of professional groups considered distinct from medicine and nursing. Some, such as dentistry and pharmacy, are not usually considered part of the 'allied health' family, but remain mainstream and informed by orthodox scientific principles, while others are viewed as 'complementary or alternative' (such as homeopathy, acupuncture or chiropractic) because they are not. Most of these professions are concerned with consulting patients, managing disease, providing diagnoses and offering treatments for ailments. What they all have in common is that none enjoy a legally sanctioned authority or scope of practice equivalent to the medical profession.

They are, or have been, constrained by legislation or regulation to a more limited scope of practice. Additions to an existing scope of practice are generally construed as constituting a form of 'advanced practice', and may even be considered grounds for recognition as a 'specialism'. Rarely are legally mandated extensions to a scope of practice agreed without a need for official approval. The legitimacy of proposed extensions may be contested or even denied. From this perspective, a profession's power to determine its own role and skill boundaries clearly influences its capacity to grow and to gain status, esteem, authority and control. What is unique about the 'allied health professions' is that they were first officially labelled as a collective by the state at a time when an emergent NHS provision was being established in the UK and occupational groups that were subordinate to medicine were needed to support medicine in managing such an ambitious scheme (Larkin, 1983; Webster, 2002; Ham, 2004).

In the UK, prior to 1948, a number of disparate healthcare occupational groups that aspired to professional status voluntarily aligned themselves to medicine through a scheme organised by the British Medical Association (BMA) in order to advance their aims through some form of official recognition (Larkin, 1983). The Board of Registration of Medical Auxiliaries offered medical recognition to 'auxiliary' professional groups in exchange for the limitation of practice and subordination to medical authority. By 1960, these groups were legally recognised as professions 'supplementary to medicine', being both established as professions and yet subordinated to the authority of medicine. State approval for this arrangement was agreed with these professions as a collective so that the government would not have to deal with a wave of disparate demands from a sea of minor self-interested groups. Thus, recognition and regulation for these professions was granted through a new regulatory body that had responsibility for overseeing a specific group of professions – those that were 'supplementary to medicine'. Therein lay the seeds of what was to become the 'allied health professions'. In the UK, dentistry and optometry already possessed their own legislative and regulatory forms of recognition, and were not therefore included as professions 'supplementary to medicine'.

Within 30 years, the professions 'supplementary' to medicine had gradually become sufficiently independent of medicine to merit the title 'allied to medicine', which, in turn, was later amended to 'allied' in recognition of yet further independence (Boyce, 2006). The 'allied health' professions thus became independent practitioners, capable of consulting patients, offering a (limited) diagnosis and initiating treatment without reliance upon medical instructions. They did not, however, become equal to medicine, and they continue to be limited in scope and authority. What processes were at work to shape the division of labour in this way? Although the 'allied health professions' appeared able to establish their legitimacy, enhance their authority and advance their professional credibility and status, they were not able to (or even aimed to) attain equality with medicine. How do we explain it? The sociology of the professions sheds light on it, and through its theoretical insights, we are able to gain a picture of what happened.

The sociology of the professions: theoretical insights

Over the last 60 years and more, the dominant theories informing the sociology of professions have changed. It is well worth examining the nature of these changes in perspective as each 'new' theoretical position added colour, depth and detail, gradually replacing the rather monotone earlier theories. It is, nevertheless, important to include the 'taxonomic' approach as it allows the reader to trace the development of thinking about the professions.

Taxonomic approach (trait and functionalist perspectives)

Initially, professions were viewed as essentially altruistic and benevolent, serving the public interest. Professionals were seen as motivated by public service rather than financial reward, and were thus a powerful force for good in society (Carr-Saunders and Wilson, 1933). Talcott Parsons (1991), an eminent sociologist, was a key exponent of functionalism and the value to society of the professions. It was felt that they should be exempt from the vagaries of a marketplace characterised by competition, as might be expected in business or industry. They were a special case, in that their altruistic service orientation and the public benefit arising from it seemed to merit recognition of a distinction between the professions and other occupations. Not only were the professions based on complex knowledge and principled ethical values, but they were above the fight when it came to the provision of services in a marketplace – matters of healthcare, for example, should not be sullied by the forces of competition in an open market. In addition, early theories proposed lists of key attributes that would be needed to enable a given occupation to merit classification as a profession (Millerson, 1964). However, by the late 1960s, it had become apparent that these theories were somewhat limited. Finding a consistent list of key attributes proved elusive and led to anomalies, such as the curious and unsatisfactory notion of 'semi-professions', a kind of purgatory in which some occupations were seemingly trapped, being neither simple occupations nor fully fledged professions (Etzioni, 1969). Indeed, nursing and the other non-medical healthcare professions (such as those that later became 'allied health') were viewed as prime examples of 'semi-professions'.

At face value, it may seem perfectly reasonable to consider professions as special types of occupation that possess particular characteristics – the six most commonly cited among them being: skill based on theoretical knowledge; required education and training; the testing of member competence; possessing/belonging to a professional body; adherence to an ethical code of conduct; and an underpinning guiding principle of altruism (Watson, 1995). Indeed, many health professionals themselves continue to identify with such an 'ideal type' approach. Yet, as later authors have pointed out, to do so would be to omit a full consideration of the relevant sociohistorical antecedents and those other factors determining success or failure in attaining such privileges. As a form of tick-box exercise, this approach would only allow a snapshot of a profession at a given point in time, and would neglect entirely any consideration of the politics of professional power and self-interest (Saks, 1983, 1995, 2010).

Professional power perspectives: asking a different question

Theorists of the professions gradually turned their attention to the importance of power in the relationships between professions and the audiences and stakeholders involved in shaping their development. While elements of differing theoretical perspectives began to draw attention to the need to consider power as a significant feature in the landscape of professionalism, one theoretical paradigm eventually came to the fore, based on the work of Max Weber (1864–1920), generally regarded as one of the founders of European sociology, and a prolific writer on political and social theory, as well as sociological method (Parkin, 2002). In the 1960s, however, it was the symbolic interactionist perspective that perhaps first questioned the utility of the trait and functionalist approaches, and presented an alternative position (Haralambos and Holborn, 2008), as unlike 'functionalist' or 'Marxian' theories, which offer a 'macro-theory' or general explanation of society, interactionism focuses more on the meanings that individuals give to their activities.

Critical of the deference shown to the professions, and the willingness to accept at face value the virtuous and ethical motives espoused by the professions themselves, symbolic interactionists sought to expose the claims as mere rhetoric designed to maintain and perpetuate professional privileges. However, the interactionist perspective was limited by its focus on micro-sociological analyses within a given workplace and its lack of consistent and compelling empirical evidence. It also failed to appreciate the broader impact of national-level structures in shaping the success or otherwise of attempts to secure the status of a profession. In common with the taxonomic approaches, it also failed to provide a sociohistorical context in its analyses. Perhaps its most important contribution, then, was to reset the underlying question and thus reframe the approach to understanding professionalisation. Instead of asking 'Is this occupation a profession?', Everett Hughes (1897–1983), a leading sociologist noted for his work on occupations and professions, posed another question, which understood 'profession' as a social value rather than a description: 'What are the circumstances in which people in an occupation attempt to turn it into a profession?' This new emphasis paved the way for what has become the most influential and empirically sound theoretical perspective: a neo-Weberian approach. However, before we turn our attention fully to it, there are some other theories that merit consideration and give greater context to the appeal of the neo-Weberian position, albeit through their limitations rather than their advances.

Marxist theory and the professions

The Marxian theoretical perspective merits attention in any consideration of the professions, albeit as a framework that has lost its lustre in recent years, particularly following the major political changes in Europe throughout the 1990s. Prominent in the 1970s and 1980s, it added important touches to the broader canvas of the professions (and draws its name from its founder, the philosopher, economist and sociologist Karl Marx [1818–83], who emphasised the importance of economic factors in determining belief and value systems) (Haralambos and Holborn, 2008). Equally concerned with power, it emphasised the role of the professions in capitalism and the class structure. Whereas Marxist and Weberian perspectives share certain points in common, they diverge over the role of professions in shaping (or being shaped by) the broader class structure in society. Both functionalist and neo-Weberian authors have been criticised for viewing the professions as somehow separate or distinct from the class structure (Larson, 1977, 1990).

In contrast, Marxist accounts focus on locating the professions within the class structure and stress the requirement that professional ideologies align with capitalist aims if professionalising strategies are to succeed. Broadly, Marxist ideology views the social structure within capitalism as comprising a form of socio-economic stratification manifest as a dominant ruling social class, which owns the means of production, and those that serve it (and are potentially exploited by it) in the form of the working class or proletariat. It is less concerned with markets (a key feature of neo-Weberian approaches) than the means of production (Saks, 1983), yet it should be acknowledged that modern industrial capitalist societies are market-based (Macdonald, 1995).

Theoretically, Marxian views are also divided in where they situate the professions in this scenario (Macdonald, 1995). As far as the health professions are concerned, Marxist analyses primarily focus upon identifying the ideological role of the middle-class professional (Navarro, 1978; Doyal, 1979). For some authors, the professions have been viewed as agents of the state, bearing a bourgeois ideology on behalf of the ruling class (a prerequisite for achieving professional status) and engaging in control and surveillance of the working class (Poulantzas, 1975; Larson, 1977; Navarro, 1978; Doyal, 1979; Esland, 1980). Physicians, for example, were said to hold control of the certification of 'legitimate' sickness and were thus empowered to maintain a workforce in the service of the ruling elite. One could not be legitimately ill unless a doctor certified it, assuring a degree of authority and control for the medical profession acting in the interests of the ruling class. For other theorists, middle-class professionals were said to bear characteristics of both the ruling and working classes, construed as both wage slaves and, at the same time, representing the interest of the bourgeoisie, where, for example, medicine controlled labour power through medical certification yet experienced increasing routinisation of work tasks (Braverman, 1974; Carchedi, 1975; Saks, 1983).

In this view, where the professions were located in both camps – capital and labour – there were some attempts at differentiation. For example, Ehrenreich and Ehrenreich (1979) saw the elite professions – the 'professional–managerial class' – as clearly serving the interests of capital, that is, as agents of the state. Navarro (1986) considered the profession of medicine to rest firmly within the capitalist class. On the other hand, for those who believed that the middle-class professions were essentially part of the proletariat (Braverman, 1974), a process of proletarianisation was already under way that would diminish the power of the professions and reduce them to the status of workers (McKinlay and Arches, 1985; Elston, 1991).

As an explanation for the loss of professional (medical) power, the proletarianisation thesis may offer some useful insights but it is considered much less convincing as part of a general theory of social change (Elston, 1991). Its key thrust is a loss of professional power due to changing work conditions and subordination to managerial control. The linked, though not explicitly Marxian, deprofessionalisation thesis also accounts for a loss in professional power, yet through a gradual rationalisation and codification of expert knowledge and a growing consumerist challenge from a more knowledgeable lay (patient) audience.

Increasingly sophisticated technological developments, and advances in areas such as artificial intelligence, may yet prove to be relevant; however, to date, the evidence in support of either thesis is sparse. Indeed, Saks, Macdonald and Parkin all provide detailed and comprehensive critiques of Marxian literature on the professions, and conclude that its explanatory power and range falls short of that offered by the neo-Weberian approach, which arguably remains the most persuasive and robust theoretical contribution to understanding the professions (Parkin, 1979; Saks, 1983; Elston, 1991; Macdonald, 1995). Broadly, then, the consensus view today is that the 'sun has now almost set' on Marxist explanations of the professions, which tend to lack substantive evidence (Macdonald, 1995: 166).

Professional knowledge: indeterminacy and technicality

Importantly for professions such as those in allied health, Johnson (1977) noted that the extent to which an occupation was liable to the effects of proletarianisation hinged upon the degree of 'indetermination' in its knowledge and skills base (Boreham, 1983; Watson, 1995). It is broadly accepted that a profession's expertise is largely based upon, or drawn from, its underlying abstract expert knowledge. Jamous and Peloille's (1970) concept of an indetermination–technicality ratio was devised to explain the necessary balance between the two required to achieve professional status. It is far from being uniquely linked to a Marxist approach (Johnson's corpus of work is not exclusively Marxist either), and its use in explaining proletarianisation should not be taken to suggest that it is limited to a Marxist analysis of the professions. In fact, the notion of a necessary blend of indeterminacy and technicality may be of particular interest to the allied health professions given the emphasis placed by them on developing a distinctive knowledge base that is sufficiently separate from medicine to justify claims to professional status, and the supposed blend of 'art' and 'science' perhaps more evident in allied health than medicine (Peloquin, 1989). Abbott (1988) also emphasised the importance of professional work, jurisdictions and expert knowledge in asserting professional status in his 'system of professions', which remains a key theoretical consideration for any study of the professions.

So, what is meant by indeterminacy and technicality in this context? Abbot related it to the range of knowledge used by professions, which spans both the 'concrete' forms and the less tangible 'abstract' types. Concrete, rational forms of professional knowledge are more widely accessible than abstract forms, more easily understood and more easily codified in a way that render them fully comprehensible to an educated lay audience. An excess of concrete, practical knowledge without formal discourse (the shrouding in mystique of complex knowledge) is regarded by clients as 'craft knowledge', something allied health professions are often keen to avoid. Why consult a physiotherapist as part of rehabilitation following a muscle injury to the leg, for example, if you can learn the techniques of massage mobilisation from a manual yourself? Clearly, 'concrete' knowledge of this type cannot form the basis of claims to expertise and professional status if anyone can master it, whether professionally trained or not.

To sustain a bid to establish or maintain professional status, it is necessary to demonstrate a form of abstract knowledge that lay people cannot easily access or grasp as it (apparently) requires special training and education – something only a professional could know and apply to solving problems. Jamous and Peloille (1970) took the view that the success of a profession hinged upon the right amount of both types of knowledge – a ratio of indeterminate (abstract) knowledge and technical (concrete) knowledge. Too much of one or the other would damage a profession's credibility and ability to sustain its privileged position within the pantheon of professions. Indeterminacy, as a form of uncertainty, requires professional judgement, based on experience, professional 'intuition' and tacit knowledge (Jamous and Peloille, 1970; Traynor, 2009). However, too much indeterminacy might mean 'other groups can claim equal or superior skill, and indeterminists lose control over their field and the ability to make predictions in it' (Traynor, 2009: 496).

Traynor goes on to point out that one further drawback to a dependence on abstraction/indeterminacy is that divisions may arise within professional subgroups over claims to aspects of indeterminacy, and even questions as to its value to the profession's work. However, allied health professionals may be interested in Traynor's (2009: 496) interpretation of Jamous and Peloille's view that those 'low down in the hierarchy of a profession' are more likely to stress 'technically based reform' than professional elites, who would emphasise indeterminacy.

Traynor's work is relevant in that it addresses the differing responses to the advent of (and ascendancy in) evidence-based practice in medicine and nursing through the 1990s and 2000s, while deploying Jamous and Peloille's thesis, which was arguably written about an era long past. Macdonald (1995) probably has the last word, in that he poses the question as to how professions can sustain a high degree of indeterminacy in their knowledge base indefinitely given the need to accept the 'primacy of scientific knowledge' in order to retain legitimacy in contemporary society. It is difficult to shroud professional knowledge in mystique in perpetuity when an emerging evidence base increasingly requires explicit and scientifically justified explanations.

Foucault, disciplinary power and 'the gaze'

Foucault's contribution to understanding the professions is significant but limited, being criticised for both 'a high level of abstractness' and a tendency to base conclusions on 'self-fulfilling arguments' drawn from a 'shaky empirical basis' (Saks, 2010: 891; see also Macdonald, 1995). Nevertheless, there are some concepts that do bring new insights to the acquisition and construction of professional knowledge, which are likely to be helpful for allied health professionals concerned to understand how professional knowledge is developed. In particular, exemplars from non-medical health professions illustrate these concepts with something approaching clarity, most notably, Nettleton's (1992) study of dentistry.

Macdonald (1995: 179) emphasised Foucault's work as philosophical rather than sociological, and thus his use of 'aspects of historical and sociological knowledge to pursue his interest in epistemology and ontology'. While Foucault's philosophical arguments are interesting, and make fascinating and compelling reading, they are not necessarily supported with evidence that may be tested for fit, in a way that would be expected or required of sociological studies. Nevertheless, the concepts of panoptic surveillance, disciplinary knowledge, the 'gaze' and the exercise of micro-powers all deserve mention for the insights they bring. On that basis, we will proceed here to explore these key concepts, with illustrative examples, without dwelling on the more abstract philosophical points raised by Foucault. For the more adventurous readers, a more detailed exposition of Foucault may be found in Macdonald's (1995) articulate and beautifully crafted text.

Foucault's key contributions have been identified as an analysis of power/knowledge, disciplinary technologies and governmentality, each of which need explanation but relate to mechanisms for regulating and controlling people and populations (Turner, 1995). Like other theorists of the period (1970s/1980s), he sought to challenge the prevalent Marxist ideology and to provide an alternative perspective to Sartre's existentialism (Eribon, 1992; Turner, 1997). Whereas Marxist notions of power were firmly rooted in the state's structures, acting in the interests of industrial capitalism (such as the police, the law and the Church), Foucault conceptualised power as something rather different (Turner, 1995). For Foucault, power was dispersed, enacted in 'micro-powers' – the mundane, day-to-day practices of professionals. Power is exerted through the 'disciplinary practices' found in everyday routines. The 'institutions of normative coercion', such as the law, religion and medicine, exert control over us but not through authoritarian control, largely because their influence is viewed as legitimate and normative. It is power that is disguised; it is manifest in discourses we willingly accept and is translated by us into acts of self-discipline in our everyday lives.

Panoptic surveillance encapsulates Foucault's view of the exercise of power, and is used by Nettleton (1992) to help explain why we, as patients, engage in such acts as tooth brushing. In the privacy of our homes (and bathrooms), where we are free to act as we choose, we nevertheless tend to brush our teeth as we are directed (advised) by our dentist. This is constituted as an act of self-policing as we obey the instruction to observe good oral hygiene by brushing our teeth every night, without being coerced into doing so. This is a 'panoptic' exercise of power, which is best explained by considering the prison design upon which it is based – the Panopticon, devised by Jeremy Bentham in the 19th century (Foucault, 1979). Unlike dungeons, where criminals in a bygone age might be cast into darkness, hidden from view, the Panopticon was designed to do the opposite – to expose the prisoner to view, to constant surveillance. Prison cells would be arranged together in a circle around a central tower, which would be visible to the inmates. The idea was that each prison cell would comprise a space bound by three walls, but where the innermost wall facing towards the central tower would be open or transparent. Prison guards would sit in the central tower and observe the inmates in their cells but, crucially, the guards would not be visible to the inmates. Thus, the prisoners would act as if they were under constant surveillance, even if the central tower was actually empty. They would engage in behaviours that were effectively self-policing, assuming that they were being observed, even when they were not being actively observed. So went the logic of the Panopticon. Nettleton's (1992) application illustrates how such authority may be translated into healthcare practices and thus reflect professional power.

Disciplinary power is dispersed, operating at the level of the individual professional. In other words, it is not an entity possessed only by elite groups, exercised in a downward direction, dominating subordinated subjects. Here, power is understood as a generative force (not a coercive force), creating knowledge through surveillance and monitoring, utilising the techniques of measurement, comparison and codification, which allows a healthcare professional to arrive at a diagnosis or treatment programme. It allows the professional to develop an explanatory discourse that constitutes the object of study – that fabricates it and perpetuates it. Knowledge generated in this way is therefore the product of a 'disciplinary regime'. It is also generated by the 'gaze' (*'le regard'*). The 'gaze' is a 'way of seeing', through which an object becomes conceptualised, constructed and thus rendered visible.

The 'gaze' helps to explain how discrete areas of the body came to be constituted and the object of disciplinary knowledge and power, and Nettleton's (1992) example of dentistry again serves to illustrate the point. Dental discourse effectively created the mouth and teeth as an object of study, as an entity separate from the rest of the body with which a profession might exclusively concern itself. Many of us might wonder why a profession would focus only on one discrete part of the body, such as the mouth and teeth (dentistry), or feet (podiatry) or eyes (optometry) – why were these parts of the body considered 'separate' enough to merit the creation of a body of knowledge about them, and an entire profession devoted exclusively to their care? It is here that Foucault's insights cast light on a dark corner. Dentistry did not emerge as a valued profession because there was a demand for it. Rather, it was created by dentistry, through an emerging knowledge of the mouth and teeth gained through a pervasive 'dental gaze' that monitored the mouths of individuals and populations. This creative disciplinary power produced new objects of knowledge, ensuring a 'normalisation' of the mouth and teeth. In the 19th century, Britain was concerned with communicable disease, with infectious diseases and epidemics, such as cholera, which were known through new insights in bacteriology to gain access to the body via the mouth. Thus, the mouth became the 'vulnerable margin' through which contaminants gained entry to the body, raising the symbolic significance of those regarded as the guardians of oral health. This enabled the surveillance of populations and thus generated disciplinary knowledge and power (Nettleton, 1992). To date, there are relatively few Foucauldian analyses of allied health professional practices and knowledge but they arguably offer fruitful additions to the literature (Borthwick, 1999; Mackey, 2007).

Finally, the notion of governmentality merits mention, though it is not for the faint-hearted. Foucault 'rejects the notion of the state as a coherent, calculating subject whose political power grows in concert with its interventions into civil society. Rather, it is viewed as an ensemble of institutions' procedures, tactics, calculations, knowledges and technologies ... the residue or outcome of governing' (Johnson, 1993: 140). It is hardly novel to recognise the wide range of interests that are brought to bear in governing, nor the contributions of its component parts, but Foucault sees it as a transition, a shift from the 'art' of government to the 'science' of government through the application and exercise of techniques of disciplinary power and surveillance. Johnson (1993: 142) considered Foucault's view of the state to reflect a 'conception of power as a social relation of tension, rather than an attribute of the subject'. For Macdonald (1995: 178), however, governmentality 'is as much a rhetorical device as an analytic concept', and really reflects little more than an 'application of modern techniques to government'.

Neo-Weberian perspectives

Perhaps the most useful theory for understanding and explaining the motives, actions and intentions of the professions is drawn from the work of Max Weber (Parkin, 1979; Saks, 1983, 2010, 2013). At its heart is an emphasis on the way professions devise strategies designed to advance their social status, capture the market for their services and actively exclude competitors while, at the same time, seeking to acquire new areas of control at the expense of others. They need to persuade both clients and the state that they merit the status and influence they seek, and that their services and skills are both desirable and essential. They are conceptualised as operating within a marketplace environment, competing with others to provide services. At first, this notion may seem irrelevant to healthcare professions, whose concern is surely the welfare and care of patients and not marketplace economics. However, on closer examination, it is clear that professions do indeed concern themselves with status, power, influence and control. They seek to establish role boundaries and control over task domains, where they retain higher-status roles and delegate lesser roles to other, often subordinate, groups. Crucially, they attempt to exclude others from access to the privileges that these roles attract, and they adopt a number of strategies to achieve this. Three key concepts inform this approach: social closure, professional dominance and the related concept of professional autonomy.

Social closure

The concept of social closure has been particularly elaborated by Parkin (1979) and Murphy (1986), and related specifically to the analysis of professionalisation by a number of authors (Freidson, 1970, 1988; Berlant, 1975; Hugman, 1991; Saks, 2010, 2012, 2014, 2016). Social closure is regarded as the process by which various social groups act to restrict access to rewards and privileges to a limited collectivity of 'eligibles' (Parkin, 1979). They do so by setting criteria, at a given point in time, by which others are excluded; this may include such markers as entry requirements to training and education, or formal, state-sanctioned registration, underpinned with legislative authority. Indeed, the most successful and enduring form of occupational closure is obtained by securing legal recognition for exclusionary practices, a characteristic feature of professional behaviour (Parkin, 1979, 1982; Larkin, 1983). Gaining the support of the state in acquiring a legal monopoly over a task domain, often associated with a defined client group, is the aim, and will ideally include penalties for those ineligible individuals who transgress the rules. Such protection may shield the profession from the marketplace, ensuring that only those within the boundaries of its recognised sphere of control have the right to determine, examine and inspect their practices. For the most part, in today's society, health professions must justify their privileges with recourse to scientific or technical rationality, as well as interpretive skills that help to ensure its knowledge is resistant to reduction (Larkin, 1983; Turner, 1985, 1995).

Intriguingly, there are two principal dimensions to social closure, known as exclusionary and usurpationary closure. Most allied health professionals will find these concepts familiar, and will recognise the examples that illustrate them. When both strategies are adopted at the same time, the term 'dual closure' applies (Parkin, 1979). Exclusionary mechanisms are enacted by occupations seeking to preserve their skills and resources (and thus avoid incursions by competitor groups), while usurpationary tactics are designed to challenge externally imposed boundaries and undermine or resist exclusion (which may involve deliberate incursions into the territory of others). Exclusion is exercised in a 'downwards' direction to ensure the subordination of less powerful competitors, while usurpation reflects an attempt at upward social mobility. Parkin (1979) identified the 'welfare semi-professions' (such as the allied health professions) as an example of those occupational groups employing both exclusionary and usurpationary methods. The use of credentials is recognised as a powerful means to protect access to key knowledge and skills, and to retain control and authority in a given sphere of practice. One only needs to look at the exemplar of rights to access and prescribe prescription-only medicines, which has only just been extended to non-medical/dental groups in recent years and yet is still not directly comparable in scope to medical prescribing (Borthwick et al, 2010).

Witz (1992) offered a further elaboration on the model of closure by introducing a fourfold distinction: exclusion, demarcation, inclusion and dual closure. Demarcation strategies are those concerned with the creation, control and negotiation of role boundaries between occupations, which may be particularly important when considering the allied health professions given their position within the healthcare hierarchy. Hugman (1991) referred to 'lateral closure' to describe much the same sort of relationship but where two professions of roughly equal power contest role boundaries, such as two allied health professions. Finally, he describes another variant, 'internal closure', which is the tendency of professions to create subgroups internally, such as 'aides' or 'assistant' grades, to whom lower-status tasks may be delegated and who are answerable and accountable to the main profession, such as is found in physiotherapy or occupational therapy. Overall, it is, of course, the more powerful professions that tend to succeed, a point that brings us to the second concept – professional dominance.

Professional dominance

Freidson first coined the term 'professional dominance', and used the medical profession to illustrate it; hence, 'medical dominance' became the most potent exemplar (Freidson, 1970, 1994; Willis, 1989, 2006). For Freidson, medical power stemmed from the legally and politically sanctioned monopoly over the organisation and control of its work, which was unique within the health division of labour. The freedom to control the content and terms of its work, the power of self-regulation, and an apparent freedom from external judgement all contributed to an unassailable position in relation to potential competitors, largely protecting medicine from boundary encroachment by less powerful groups (Freidson, 1988, 1994, 2001). His point was that medicine enjoyed an authority that extended beyond self-regulation and control; it involved power over other professions, notably, a degree of control over the allied health and nursing professions. At the time, non-medical professions were excluded from certain key roles, functions and skills, such as making a medical diagnosis, prescribing medicines or undertaking invasive surgery (Freidson, 1988). Willis (1989) also arrived at similar conclusions, drawing a distinction between authority, autonomy and sovereignty, in which the medical profession alone occupied the enviable position of possessing all three forms of control. Autonomy is seen as self-regulation, authority as control over other professions (such as allied health and nursing) and sovereignty as power within wider society, where medical accounts are accepted as authoritative and legitimate (Willis, 1989, 2006). Elston (1991) established a clear analytic distinction between the concepts of 'dominance' and 'autonomy', which she felt had too often been used interchangeably. Dominance she saw as medicine's authority over others, which could be divided into social authority (control over the actions of others, for example, though giving instructions on treatment) and cultural authority, which was the 'probability that medical definitions of reality and medical judgements will be accepted as valid and true' (Elston, 1991: 61).

These concepts were largely established in the 1970s and early 1980s, and things have changed in many ways; however, medicine is still the most powerful healthcare profession and continues to exercise considerable social, cultural and political influence, which is clearly not matched by nursing or the allied health professions. Even at the time, Larkin (1983: 8) considered the concept of medical dominance to be excessively one-sided, suggesting that it was 'over muscular' and guilty of a 'zero sum conflict'. He argued cogently that medicine should not be portrayed as the sole perpetrator of tyrannical dominance, with nursing and the allied health professions as innocent victims. For Larkin, the paramedical professions (by which he meant allied health and nursing) were equally capable of adopting exclusionary tactics but less successful in achieving their desired outcomes.

Larkin (1983) suggested an even clearer concept that captured the competitive strategies deployed by a range of differing professions – 'occupational imperialism'. Occupational imperialism denotes the strategies and tactics adopted by each occupation to shape the division of labour to its advantage. The tactics employed involve poaching skills from other professional groups or delegating skills to lesser groups in a bid to secure income, status and control. It is striking how such a dynamic appears to fit closely to the reality of the allied health professions: operating in the shadow of a more powerful medical profession; competing with each other for control over certain roles, tasks and boundaries of practice; while also establishing an internal hierarchy of aides and assistants to whom the 'dirty work' may be given. The constant tension that this process suggests, particularly when considering the health division of labour and its clear hierarchy, is captured in Abbott's (1988) 'system of professions' and most clearly in his conception of 'jurisdictional disputes', in which professions actively contest spheres of work – jurisdictions in the workplace. For Abbott, workplace role and boundary disputes are the key source of tension between professions. Each seeks advancement through extending role boundaries, assuming more prestigious roles from which to gain status, better remuneration and societal esteem.

Hugman (1991) referred to these sought-after roles as 'virtuoso roles', which require special skill and high levels of knowledge, and that command particular respect and reverence. Abbott's focus on the importance of role jurisdictions underpinned with special knowledge is convincing in its logic, though the suggestion that, in its entirety, it is part of a wider interacting system is perhaps less obviously so. Macdonald (1995) is sceptical and finds it to be rather similar to functionalism, which omits the actors' motives so central to Weberian analyses. Macdonald (1995) does, however, assign great importance to the concept of the 'professional project' developed by Larson (1977), and it fully merits consideration here, for it draws together many of the strands that exist within the neo-Weberian framework.

The professional project

Magali Larson (1977) constructed the concept of a 'professional project', which draws together Weber's views on social stratification and the use of credentials as opportunities for income in a market-based society with Freidson's work on the way professions seek to establish and maintain professional autonomy, status and prestige through the support of social and political 'elites' (Macdonald, 1995). Central to her concept is the recognition that specialist skills and expertise do not, in themselves, result automatically in higher social status or market control. They are fought for and won (and maintained and expanded) through the actions comprising the 'professional project'. This is a collective project within a profession, yet, intriguingly, the aims and plans of a group are not always evident or intended by all of its members (Larson, 1977; Macdonald, 1995). This is an important corollary as it reinforces the idea that the professional project is not simply designed to achieve a given strategic outcome, at which point it may be set aside; rather, it is a constant, ongoing process that must adapt to wider political and societal change if it is to continue to be successful. Access to university degree credentials, state recognition through licensing or registration, the royal college or chartered status of professional bodies, and a unique and exclusive knowledge base and skills within the healthcare market are all familiar elements to allied health professionals and form part of the professional project that each has established and constantly strives to maintain, expand and grow. Macdonald (1995) is clearly an advocate of Larson's professional project, and less enamoured of Abbott's 'system of professions', yet concedes that drawing on the latter to add to the former has merit, in that 'what needs to be added to Larson's formulation is the recognition that a profession does not merely mark out its domain in a bargain with the state; it has to fight other occupations for it, not only at the time, but before and after as well' (Macdonald, 1995: 33).

On balance, it is the neo-Weberian approach to the professions that offers the greatest explanatory power and understanding not only of what professions do, but also of what motivates them to do it. It is no coincidence that the leading academics and researchers in the field of the sociology of the professions in the contemporary world continue to argue for the pre-eminence of neo-Weberian theoretical frameworks, as exemplified by the substantial and hugely impressive corpus of work by Saks (1983, 1995, 1999, 2003, 2010, 2014, 2015, 2016, 2017, 2018).

Bourdieu: symbolic capital and symbolic violence

Pierre Bourdieu may have recommended that contemporary use of the terms 'profession' and 'professionalism' be 'abandoned because they are stereotypes' (Olgiati, 2010: 808) but this does not mean that his work has no further relevance to the study of professions; far from it. His work is concerned with power struggles in the social world, and how advantage is secured and reproduced. These power struggles occur within a 'social space', where individuals are defined by their relative positions within the space, which, in turn, becomes a 'field of forces', that is, a form of objective power relations that impact on everyone who enters the field (Bourdieu, 1985). What are the forces that are 'active' in the field? They are constituted as the key assets or resources that confer power – forms of 'capital'. For Bourdieu, this includes economic capital, social capital (important social networks and relationships), cultural capital (forms of knowledge that are recognised as legitimate) and symbolic capital (prestige, reputation and renown) (Bourdieu, 1985; Jenkins, 2002). Capital, in its various forms, constitutes a valuable potential resource that, once attained, confers considerable social advantage on those who possess it. The field of power is the dominant field, the origin of hierarchical power relations that gives structure to every other field (Jenkins, 2002). Those that possess power control the means to access power, thus creating a cycle that reinforces the power that they possess (the 'circle of symbolic reproduction').

Symbolic capital (prestige, status and renown) is a source of power attained by dominant groups in such a way as to successfully persuade others to accept it as legitimate, as obvious (Bourdieu, 1985; Jenkins, 2002; King et al, 2018). In achieving this outcome – that power is exercised in a way that is considered legitimate, as taken-for-granted – the exercise of power is concealed (Bourdieu and Passeron, 1990). One facet of this that will resonate clearly with allied health professionals is the way in which professional titles of prestige are controlled. Prestigious titles are symbolic capital; they are desirable and sought after, and they confer high status on those who possess them. Examples within healthcare might be 'consultant', until recently considered to be a title reserved for the highest rank of medical practitioner, or 'surgeon'. The latter title enjoys a legal legitimation in the UK and Australia but variants of it may be used by other, non-medical, practitioners, who have, as a result, been subject to 'symbolic violence'. Symbolic violence describes the way in which claims to symbolic capital by less powerful groups are devalued through subtle expressions of aggression as a means to protect, in this case, the scarcity value of the title 'surgeon', even when the roles and tasks carried out by the 'other' may involve surgery. At stake is the legitimate power to name, to assign title and to have it socially and even legally recognised. For Bourdieu (1985: 733), it is 'the symbolic scarcity of the title in the space of the names of the professions that tends to govern the rewards of the occupation (and not the relationship between the supply and demand for a particular form of labour)'. For example, where medical professionals oppose the use of titles by other, non-medical, practitioners, such as nurses or allied health professionals, they use the compelling logic of legitimacy, obscuring the concealed symbolic violence within it (Bourdieu and Passeron, 1990; Borthwick et al, 2015). They may argue, with some logic, that most people (patients) would automatically assume that any healthcare practitioner using the title of 'consultant' or 'surgeon' (or, worse still, both together) would not only be medically qualified, but also be a very senior medical professional (Borthwick et al, 2015). The implication is that non-medically qualified health practitioners should not be so disingenuous as to use such titles. Crucially, for Bourdieu (1985: 733), 'it is not the relative value of the work that determines the value of the name, but the institutionalised value of the title that can be used as a means of defending or maintaining the value of the work'. Titles, therefore, are rather more important than we tend to assume.

Sociology offers a rich and compelling range of explanatory frameworks and theoretical constructs that help shed light on the professions. It allows practitioners to perhaps step beyond their own 'taken-for-granted' assumptions and consider a more critical, analytical approach to studies of the professions and those that inhabit them. This Introduction aims to provide readers an accessible insight into current sociological theory, and how it may be applied to their own professions. It also provides a grounding in theory that informs the chapters that follow.

Book overview

This book is structured to provide a detailed exploration of the concept of the allied health collective, and then to illustrate the allied health professions through different stages of professionalisation. We recognise that within the heterogeneous collective of the allied health professions, they are at different stages of their own professional project. While the most commonly recognised allied health professions, such as physiotherapy, optometry, podiatry and radiography, have long and established histories, new professions continue to emerge. Others have created an internal division of labour through the introduction of support workers; furthermore, we see the growth of new interdisciplinary roles and formalised processes of task-sharing that we have termed 'post-professionalism'.

To explore these concepts, we compare a range of purposively selected case studies of allied health professions and emerging occupations in Australia and the UK. The case studies have been selected to illustrate specific issues relevant to the stage of professionalisation and their identity within the allied health profession collective. Through this interprofessional and international comparison, we draw on the theory of the sociology of the professions to identify and describe: the different stages of evolution through which the allied health professions may progress to achieve their professional project; the strategies they use to compete and evolve; the success of those strategies in achieving their professional project; and the impact of those strategies on the professions.

Chapter 1 examines the concept of allied health as a confederation of constituent professions. We examine: the way that different jurisdictions define the allied health collective; the rationale for those groupings; and the impact of inclusion (or otherwise) of the groupings on the individual professional project of specific allied health professions. Concepts that will be explored include the considerations around a heterogeneous group of occupations attempting to work together to achieve a single professional project (Boyce, 2001, 2006; Kreindler et al, 2012). Chapter 1 also explores the international contexts of the allied health professions and the relevance of the specific comparisons between Australia and the UK.

A glaring omission from the allied health literature is the analysis of diversity, particularly given the highly feminised nature of the allied health disciplines. To start to address this omission and establish an important context for the remaining text, Chapter 2 is dedicated to an analysis of diversity within the allied health professions, including the intersectional relationships between gender, class, ethnicity, interprofessionality and cultural competence.

The following chapters are structured around various stages of professional evolution and maturity to explore the processes of negotiation that the allied health professions have had to undergo to achieve their current positions. The well-established and more mature allied health professions have had to negotiate their professional boundaries with the state and the medical profession. In many ways, it is these early disputes and negotiations that are responsible for shaping the modern health workforce and the allied health division of labour. This early development is explored in detail in Chapter 3 using the examples of optometry and radiography.

In contrast, newly emerging allied health professions at the end of the 20th century and start of the 21st century have been able to access a far more straightforward pathway to achieve their professional project. Newly emerging occupations that meet a series of minimum professional standards face limited opposition from the state and minimal, if any, intervention from the medical profession. Their primary challenge is achieving professional closure and convincing large (mostly state) funding bodies to recognise and purchase their services, effectively achieving professional closure. Chapter 4 draws on the examples of the professionalisation of ODPs, pedorthists and developmental educators (DEs) to examine the pathway to professionalism in the late 20th and early 21st centuries. These examples illustrate potential pathways that can be adopted for successful professionalisation by other occupational groups.

Allied health professionals have successfully devolved several aspects of their work to a growing support workforce, such as allied health assistants. These roles are becoming increasingly standardised in terms of training, titles, recognition and regulation. These occupations are often seen as transitional roles rather than aspiring professions in their own right, and may occupy an interdisciplinary space; however, there is evidence of growth and extended scope within these disciplines, such as the expansion of occupational therapy assistant (OTA) roles into assistant practitioners. Chapter 5 draws on the examples of OTAs and podiatry assistants to examine the development and growth of the support workforce in allied health, and the considerations for the allied health professions.

Few allied health professions have successfully achieved recognised specialisms. The medical profession particularly and the nursing profession to a lesser extent have both been successful in achieving internal divisions of labour through state-recognised specialisations. While many allied health professions recognise 'special interests' and endorse specialist areas of practice, few of these specialisms are formally recognised by the state or attract a higher level of professional recognition through higher roles and reimbursement. The two notable exceptions to this are the practice of psychology and podiatry. Chapter 6 explores the development of podiatric surgery as a state-registered allied health specialisation, and the negotiations with the state and the medical profession that shaped it.

One relatively unique feature of the allied health professions is the extent of interdisciplinary and transdisciplinary working across the continuum of professionalisation. These trans- and interdisciplinary relationships can be negotiated at a team or institutional level; however, they are also formalised into recognised training structures and professional hierarchies, particularly in the fields of diabetes education, mental health and in generic assessment and case management roles, such as with the National Disability Insurance Scheme (NDIS) in Australia and with intermediate and transitional care for older people in the UK. In Chapter 7, we explore these post-professional roles in more detail, and the implications of these roles for the allied health professions generally.

The concluding chapter considers the policy and practice implications of the preceding chapters. The second half of the chapter revisits the concept of the allied health collective to consider the definition, value and meaning of this collective in the 21st-century workforce. Considering the influences on allied health over the past century, we speculate about possible future directions for the professions.

The heterogeneity of the professions and international variations mean that the terms speech pathology and speech and language therapy have been used interchangeably. Similarly, we recognise that allied health professions use a range of terms to refer to their service users, including patients, service users and clients. These terms have been used interchangeably according to the context in which they are applied.

ONE

The allied health collective

This chapter examines the concept of allied health as a collective comprised of constituent professional groupings. Here, we describe the development of the allied health professions over the past century from the perspective of both the development of individual professions and the emergence of allied health under medical hegemony. Concepts that will be explored include considerations around a heterogeneous group of occupations attempting to work together to achieve a single professional project. We also examine the international health and social care organisational and policy contexts and the importance of the various regulatory frameworks.

What are the 'allied health professions'?

The allied health professions are distinct from the medical and nursing professions in numerous ways. Collectively, allied health professions comprise approximately one third of the total health workforce. Due to large jurisdictional variations in inclusion in the allied health collective, as well as challenges in capturing allied health workforce data, the exact numbers and scale of the allied health professions vary widely and are difficult to determine accurately (Olson, 2012; Nancarrow et al, 2017).

Unlike medicine and nursing, which have strong brand recognition, large individual professional size, internal hierarchies, recognised specialisms and, importantly, a strong political voice, the allied health professions are a confederation of independent disciplines, each of varying size and focusing on a niche area of practice. Allied health professions face the dual challenge of negotiating their discrete professional territory within the boundaries of the allied health collective, while attempting to achieve recognition and a voice alongside their larger medical and nursing counterparts.

The established allied health professions share with nursing a period of growth in the 20th century that was subject to medical dominance, largely characterised by one of three modes of domination: subordination, limitation and exclusion (Turner, 1985). For Turner, these related directly to the extent to which the 'paramedical' professions were subject to medical authority in the form of direct instructions in practice (thus depriving the profession of autonomy), by permitting autonomy within a limited jurisdiction (to a discrete body part, such as in dentistry, or a distinct therapeutic technique, such as in pharmacy) or, indeed, by rejection of the scientific legitimacy of its claimed knowledge base (as in chiropractic). Allied health professions reflect Turner's typology, in that they are built upon a limited area of practice, either confined to a specific part of the body (audiology) or to a specialised technique (sonography), though it is less clear whether this is due to medical dominance (reactive), the occupation of a jurisdictional vacancy (proactive) or both (Turner, 1985).

A key feature that differentiates allied health from nursing and medicine is the collective and poorly circumscribed groups of individual disciplines that allied health can include. As a result of their individual small sizes, allied health services are often seen and managed collectively within organisations and by purchasers and funders (Boyce, 1996; The Coalition of Health Professionals, 2001). One of the challenges associated with the confederation of allied health professions is the lack of unity of voice. Up to 200 different professions have been labelled as 'allied health' professions (Olson, 2012). These professions vary greatly in size, scope, status and skills (Nancarrow et al, 2017), which means that it is impossible for health care funders and decision-makers to consult individually with every actual (or prospective) allied health profession (Olson, 2012).

Abbott (1988) proposed that professional authority is dependent on achieving successful jurisdictional demands. This process is determined in a power struggle, where the number and quality of knowledge resources in the profession and its individual members is crucial. The allied health collective creates a single point of negotiation or discussion for the allied health group. Similarly, Freidson (1970) proposes that professions gain recognition through their alliance with powerful elites. While allied health professions have historically achieved this on a profession-by-profession basis, it also makes sense that the allied health collective will need to court the state for benefits and recognition, and a larger united voice will support that goal (Larkin, 1983). However, as we outline in Chapter 2, the allied health professions also face interprofessional tensions that challenge their own position within the hierarchy of the allied health collective.

Another relatively unique attribute of the allied health professions is that the constituent professions have continued to emerge. There is a core 'stable' of recognised professions, such as physiotherapy, podiatry/chiropody, optometry/opticians, occupational therapy and speech language therapy/pathology, many of which existed (or were emerging) at the start of the 20th century. Several new allied health professions are now recognised as a result of changing societal needs, changing demographic profiles, new technologies and new approaches to care. While not all jurisdictions recognise the emergent allied health professions, and not all emergent professions identify as allied health, the allied health professions have demonstrated that they are nimble in their ability to develop or recognise niche areas and establish a recognised professional identity in this space. New allied health professions include sonographers, audiologists, exercise physiologists, rehabilitation counsellors and DEs. We discuss the process through which new professions can emerge in Chapter 4.

At the same time, doctors and nurses have established new specialisms, often endorsed through internal hierarchies. However, unlike the allied health professions, which are often in competition with each other for patients, the internal hierarchies of the nursing and medical professions act to strengthen their professions rather than create internal competition.

Despite the large numbers of allied health professionals, little has been written about allied health service providers collectively. Instead, the literature is fragmented into descriptions of allied health and, within that, the multiple, poorly defined and contextually dependent disciplines from which they are constituted (Boyce, 1996; Nicholls, 2018). Sociological and historic analyses of the allied health professions individually and collectively are extremely limited. While the term 'allied health' is now relatively widely used in Anglo–American countries, it has a relatively recent inception. Additionally, membership to the allied health collective is poorly defined and varies according to jurisdiction, funding body and regulator.

The first use of the term 'allied health' is attributed to a 1966 meeting of the deans of 13 universities in the US that trained health professionals (Olson, 2012). The term 'allied health' was proposed to describe essential health services that are not medicine, dentistry or nursing. Shortly afterwards, the Allied Health Professions Personnel Training Act 1966 was introduced in the US, which was supported by over a decade of substantial increases in funding for allied health training and education. According to Olson, the use of the term 'allied health' was not popular unless it was associated with access to federal funding. Since then, the term has been widely adopted; however, there is still no consistent definition.

In the UK, the formation of the NHS was formative in the development of the allied health professions. In 1949, a committee chaired by Zachary Cope (known as the Cope Committee) was established to investigate the training models of, supply of, demand for and qualifications of the professions then known as 'medical auxiliaries' employed in the NHS, which included radiographers, chiropodists, physiotherapists, laboratory technicians, dieticians, almoners and speech and language therapists (Larkin, 1983). Following much debate on the processes and recommendations of the Cope Committee, the Professions Supplementary to Medicine Act 1960 was introduced for the registration of all the aforementioned disciplines, except speech and language therapists, who withdrew during the course of the Bill. The Council of the Professions Supplementary to Medicine presided over these (and other) disciplines until it was restructured as the Health Professions Council (HPC) in April 2002 (Department of Health, 2000) and subsequently as the HCPC. Until this time (and even beyond), the term 'professions allied to medicine' was commonly used to describe allied health professionals in the UK, though there is little documentation on the collective history of allied health prior to this time.

Now, in the UK NHS, all recognised allied health professions are registered with and regulated by the HCPC. At the start of 2020, the NHS formally recognised 14 allied health professions: art therapists, diagnostic radiographers, drama therapists, dietitians, music therapists, occupational therapists, ODPs, orthoptists, osteopaths, paramedics, physiotherapists, prosthetists/orthotists, speech and language therapists, and therapeutic radiographers.

Intriguingly, the move into the broad fold of allied health by osteopathy marks a shift in its status from an 'alternative' medical practice largely excluded from mainstream legitimacy to an accepted and state-regulated profession (Turner, 1985, 1995). Although it had already secured a degree of legitimation through its own Act of Parliament in 1993, its inclusion within allied health may have afforded it greater integration within mainstream healthcare. It remains to be seen if other professions that occupy the 'complementary and alternative' space may yet become recognised as allied health professions in the UK, such as chiropractic, acupuncture, homeopathy or medical herbalism (Saks, 1995, 1999).

The early history of allied health in Australia is poorly documented, though Boyce (1996) suggests that the first National Allied Health Conference in Australia in 1992 was a pivotal time for cementing allied health identity. The Australian Council of Allied Health Professionals, an overarching body representing allied health professional organisations nationally, was established in the mid-1990s. This group was subsequently renamed the 'Health Professionals Council of Australia' in 1998 (Health Professions Council of Australia, 1998) and, more recently, 'Allied Health Professions Australia', which collectively represented 21 professional groups in 2020. Several other state and territory groups formed for lobbying purposes and to support the specific needs of professionals and patients. For example the Coalition of Health Professionals (New South Wales) formed in response to the introduction of 'preferred provider' purchasing models by health insurance companies (The Coalition of Health Professionals, 2001). Similar models evolved in other states. These groups collectively provide the constituent disciplines with the bargaining strength and political lobbying power that their individual small sizes do not allow. The needs and interests of specific groups, including rural allied health providers and indigenous allied health workers, are supported through specific lobbying groups, such as Services for Australian Rural and Remote Allied Health (see: https://sarrah.org.au) and Indigenous Allied Health Australia (see: https://iaha.com.au).

Allied health in Australia was fragmented by profession, state and different levels of professional recognition until 2010, when the Australian National Registration and Accreditation Scheme (NRAS) was established to provide national registration, initially for ten health professions: chiropractic, dental practice, medicine, nursing and midwifery, optometry, osteopathy, physiotherapy, podiatry, and psychology (Carlton, 2017). In 2012, four additional professions were included: Aboriginal and Torres Strait Islander health practice, Chinese medicine, medical radiation practice, and occupational therapy. There are several other recognised allied health professions that are not part of NRAS, and every Australian state, organisation and funding body has adopted it's own definition of allied health.

Despite the established use of the term 'allied health', the concept remains elusive. The confederated nature of the professions means that there is little uniting them except their exclusion from the nursing and medical division hierarchy. They differentiate themselves from complementary and alternative medicine practitioners, largely on philosophical grounds, including adherence to the medical orthodox view. However, as complementary and alternative medicine practitioners increasingly attempt to professionalise, these differences are diminishing, as reflected by the shift in identity of osteopathy from complementary medicine to an allied health profession noted earlier. As the following chapters show, the context for the development of the allied health professions is important.

The centralised model of the NHS acts as a large monopoly employer of all allied health professions. The allied health professions need to comply with their individual professional regulatory requirements and in return receive legislative protection of their titles. This has created a market stability around the allied health professions that is not evident in other English-speaking countries. In particular, there has been a great deal of stability of the types of allied health professions recognised in the NHS. Unlike the more devolved healthcare market in Australia, which enables a certain degree of entrepreneurship in the development of new professions, the NHS provides few opportunities for new professions to emerge.

Apart from their delineated titles, the NHS allied health professions are employed on a common pay scale (Agenda for Change) and measured against equivalent competencies (Department of Health, 2001). This model creates the potential for a large amount of internal flexibility and task transfer within that framework, though, in reality, it is not clear that this occurs. In contrast, the more pluralistic markets (and more open market environments) of Australasia and North America create opportunities for the development of new professions that have convinced society of the need for their services and created a sufficient haven to protect and reward those roles, often without state protection.

The nature of allied health profession work

The medical profession and nursing are large occupation groups with a generalist base that focuses on the whole body and overall health. It is here, perhaps, that Turner's (1985) concept of 'limitation' offers a clearer differentiation between them and the allied health professions given the confined arena of practice notable in so many allied health professions, such as optometry, podiatry, pharmacy or radiography. Medicine and nursing's large size and broad scope make way for internal hierarchies and specialisations. In the medical profession, up to 50 different specialities can be recognised depending on the jurisdiction, such as surgery, psychiatry, radiography, paediatrics, haematology and ophthalmology (Medical Board of Australia, 2018; British Medical Association, 2020; Canadian Medical Association, 2020). Specialisation within the medical profession generally involves substantial additional training and membership of a recognised college, and is associated with increased recognition and rewards (Nancarrow and Borthwick, 2005).

Within the medical profession, the status of different types of speciality varies according to the types of activity (Shortell, 1974). Tasks requiring less skill or those with less esteem are more likely to be delegated to others. The complexity of work also forms a framework for understanding its status (Abbott, 1981), where 'routine' or less complex work is more likely to be managed by the lower-status profession, whereas more complex or 'less routine' tasks are more likely to be referred to the specialist practitioner (Freidson, 1970). Abbott (1981) takes the concept of intra-professional status further, proposing that status is a function of 'professional purity', in which the highest-status professionals deal with more highly processed issues and problems, which have had the 'human complexity' removed by others. Conversely, the lowest-status work involves the greatest human complexity. Larkin (1983) suggests that the divisions in medical work are the product of technological innovation, rather than intra-professional boundaries, and uses the example of the development of radiographers to allow the medical application of X-rays.

The nursing profession has also developed internal hierarchies, recognising advanced practice roles in many jurisdictions and fields (Gardner et al, 2016; King et al, 2017b; Parker and Hill, 2017). These internal hierarchies generally require additional training and, in turn, are associated with greater recognition and rewards.

In contrast, the allied health professions have each evolved around a narrow (niche) scope of practice, around a particular philosophy of care (for example, occupation and occupational therapy), body part (for example, podiatry/chiropody and the foot) or technology (for example, sonographers, optometrists and pedorthists). The attributes of the allied health professions have some overlap and, in some cases (for example, the musculoskeletal professions), competing approaches. A further differentiator of the allied health professions is that they tend to function along different parts of the continuum of care, from prevention to rehabilitation and maintenance (Philip, 2015).

These areas of niche practice are an important differentiator for the allied health professions; however, they also explain the need for them to work collectively. The allied health professions do not have a monopoly on a broad repertoire of skills and whole-body knowledge, as could be said of the medical profession. Instead, they have adopted niche or virtuoso roles, or have aligned themselves with specific body parts, philosophies or approaches to care that, in themselves, preclude the fully autonomous practice of medicine as we currently understand it. This is important because the allied health professions have lacked the critical size and breadth of work to develop an internal division of labour; instead, new skills and tasks may become adopted as the repertoire of the whole occupational group but do not generally form part of a new, hierarchical division of labour within the allied health occupation group.

This is not to say that many allied health professions do not recognise areas of special interest or advanced scope of practice (Saxon et al,

2014), but there are limited organisational and regulatory structures to recognise them. For instance, Agenda for Change created pathways for allied heath consultants and extended scope practitioners; however, where they exist, these are roles that are locally developed and lack a standardised and externally recognised title (McPherson et al, 2004). Conversely, as the case study of the diabetes educator in Chapter 7 illustrates, when new roles are adopted by the nursing profession (such as diabetes education), this can become part of an advanced role for nurses, attracting increased rewards and recognition.

The size and hierarchical structures of the nursing and medical professions enable them to embrace a wide range of specialities and skill structures within their division of labour. This provides a level of flexibility for those professions to respond to changing patient, political and organisational needs, and to adopt new evidence by expanding their repertoire to create new specialisations, while delegating lower-status or less-skilled tasks to other workers within the same division of labour. In so doing, the professions maintain overall control of their skill repertoire. The same is untrue for the allied health professions. Instead, as Chapter 4 illustrates, one response to new workforce needs is the emergence of new, autonomous occupations that become allied health professions.

An additional player worth discussing in the health sphere in the context of allied health is complementary medicine. In many ways, the development of the complementary and alternative therapies has a great deal of synergy with the allied health professions. Both allied health professionals and complementary therapists have been through a similar journey of professionalisation after long, and sometimes well-organised, pre-profession stages (Larkin, 1983). Osteopathy, in particular, was perceived to be a threat to the medical profession but, through a high level of organisation and state intervention, achieved professionalisation (registration) in Australia and the UK (Baer, 2009), and is now considered an allied health profession.

Coulter and Willis (2007: 215) describe the philosophical features that help define and differentiate complementary and alternative medicine from orthodox allopathic medicine:

> Where orthodox, allopathic medicine represents a relatively unified paradigm of knowledge about illness and health as well as treatments based on that knowledge. To a considerable extent, internal rules have emerged for resolving debates about treatments relying on the tenets of evidence-based medicine, the Cochrane collaboration and

so on. Yet the same cannot be said of CAM [complementary and alternative medicine].

Like allied health, the complementary and alternative medicine disciplines lack a unifying theory or paradigm to which all disciplines adhere. Coulter and Willis recognise that complementary and alternative medicine practitioners from within the same discipline may use treatment approaches from a range of theories or philosophies, some of which may be internally inconsistent. Instead, they propose that the unifying feature of the complementary and alternative medicine disciplines is their adoption of the principle of 'vitalism', which is 'the acceptance of all living organisms as sustained by a vital force that is both different from, and greater than, physical and chemical forces' (Coulter and Willis, 2007: 215).

This is a useful distinction because a further defining feature of the allied health professions could be seen to be their adherence to and adoption of the orthodox, Western medical principles about knowledge of illness and health. An alternative and more contemporary (but perhaps cynical) suggestion is that of managerial uniformity, in which as long as the profession functions within centrally endorsed rules for practice, causes no harm and can convince the public to purchase its services, there is little scrutiny of its practice.

The international context of allied health

While many allied health professions have ancient origins, and some may share similarities with other traditional workforces, the modern allied health workforce is firmly situated within a Western, post-industrial and largely English-speaking context. Much of the sociology of the professions is positioned ethnocentrically from a British/American perspective (Macdonald, 1995), and, further, assumes a homogeneity between the UK and the US, or, as one commentator proposes, the 'Ambrit fallacy' (Littler, 1978). The Ambrit fallacy refers to a tendency to draw sociological conclusions based on a mistaken conflation of US and UK societies. Studies of the professions largely commence with the UK's Industrial Revolution. Few analyses of the sociology of the professions explicitly examine the role that the state and political structures have had on the evolution of the professions. Instead, they assume that the context in which the profession is studied (largely the UK context) is the normative frame for analysis.

MacDonald (1995) identifies several weaknesses of the ethnocentrism of the sociology of the professions, including: that the terms 'professional' and 'professionalisation' are strongly bound up with the English language (Torstendahl, 1990); that existing frameworks are too bound up with the Anglo–American framework to cope with the comparative social history that the profession now requires; that theories of the professions are assumed to have universal applicability, when much of the data is derived from narrow, English-speaking samples; and that the notion of the professions is heavily rooted in industrialised nations. The cultural heritage of the allied health professions is almost completely ignored in the literature; however, the few texts that do exist (Larkin, 1983; Willis, 1983) assume a predominantly British heritage. This is partly due to the lack of published data, the large and inconsistently defined numbers of professions, and the numerous jurisdictions in which allied health practitioners work and are regulated.

It is notable that allied health is predominantly seen in the context of higher-income, Western nations. The uptake of allied health professions in low-income, Asian and African nations has been much less consistent. An analysis by Chen (2001) on the challenges faced by low-income countries in the adoption of the Western medical model may help to explain the distribution of allied health professionals globally. Chen describes the evolution of the health system in the Peoples' Republic of China (PRC) for the three decades from 1949 under Mao Zedong until the market reforms from the late 1970s. Post-war China faced enormous population health challenges, including infectious disease, epidemics and poor nutrition and sanitation, which resulted in high rates of infant mortality and very low life expectancy. The health workforce at the time predominantly comprised traditional Chinese medicine practitioners and herbalists, who lacked the public health skills and training to meet the needs of the population. The dominant Western medical model was rejected by Mao Zedong as a solution to the population health challenges for several reasons: the long and expensive training models; the focus on individual, curative models rather than population health and prevention; and the high dependence on technology (Wilenski, 1976; Chen, 2001). Chen (2001) suggests that the medical model was only appropriate for industrialised countries that had essentially undergone a demographic transition and had reasonable life expectancy, and where nutrition and sanitation were sufficiently developed (see also Larsen and Hodne, 1988).

Instead, the PRC introduced a model that trained local practitioners who could be mobilised in a much shorter training time and whose interventions were labour-intensive rather than using capital-intensive medical technologies. Health workforce delivery was based on the principles of prevention and supported by public health infrastructure;

supporting the workers and peasants, and integrating traditional Chinese and Western medicine, health work was to be delivered into communities through 'mass movements' (Chen, 2001). Mass movements were large-scale public health campaigns that combined the rapid training of front-line workers with targeted messaging about specific health issues and mass population engagement. Most rural healthcare was delivered through locally trained 'barefoot doctors': part-time peasants and farmers who received some training from medically trained physicians and were able to deliver some basic care, support and coordination of services close to home. After the introduction of market reforms in China, the barefoot doctors were replaced by village doctors, who require a minimum of three years education (Hu et al, 2017).

Today, China has a multi-tiered medical training system, with Western-trained medical doctors predominantly employed in large hospitals (not in primary healthcare), and primary healthcare delivered by village doctors or equivalent trained practitioners (Hsieh and Tang, 2019). Allied health is not a mainstream component of the Chinese health workforce, though traditional Chinese medicine is still an integral component of Chinese healthcare. The coexistence of traditional and orthodox (Western) health practices is not uncommon, and is recognised as an important strategy to maintain healthy populations, particularly in low- and middle-income countries (World Health Organization, 2013).

The challenges of introducing an allied health workforce in low- and middle-income countries is illustrated through a contemporary Nigerian example of attempts to credential traditional bonesetters to become orthopaedic technicians (Onyemaechi et al, 2020). Bonesetters are a traditional workforce, often inheriting the role and training through their family lineage or as a 'gift from God'. They enjoy high levels of support from their local communities and are the first choice of treatment for the majority of bone fractures in rural Nigerian communities (Onyemaechi et al, 2020). Their widespread uptake arises from their long-standing role and importance in their communities, which pre-dates the introduction of Western orthopaedic interventions. They are seen to be affordable, be easily accessible and provide a faster service than other alternatives while aligning with the sociocultural beliefs of the population (Onyemaechi et al, 2020). In many cases, there are no alternative providers available. However, their lack of formal training and wide variations in practice mean that outcomes are varied, and adverse events are not uncommon. In recognition of the value of the role of the traditional bonesetters but also the risks arising from their lack of training, there is a move to introduce the credentialed training of traditional bonesetters. This requires an unusual level of collaboration with and support from the orthodox orthopaedic practitioners; however, there is acceptance of the need for training by the bonesetters, in part, due to the increased credibility and recognition that standardised training will provide their workforce.

These lessons are valuable to both understanding why allied health has had a relatively slow uptake in many low- and middle-income countries, and appreciating the skills embedded within traditional workforces. Chapter 4 discusses emerging professions, in which traditional, vocationally trained workforces or new occupational groups that address a niche area of practice have professionalised to become allied health professions. The route to becoming an allied health profession is dependent on: public recognition and valuing of the occupational group; organised systems of formalised and credentialed training; and opportunities for regulation (which may be state-run or profession-led). Such pathways may be available to support the professionalisation pathway of existing workforces in low- and middle-income countries in order to ensure some standardisation of practice and quality assurance processes.

While there are strong trends and themes that unite the allied health professions internationally, particularly in terms of their professional identity, there are several important sociopolitical differences in their implementation that have shaped their development and evolution. Of importance are the regulatory and organisational frameworks. As we show in Chapter 4, the NHS has conflated state recognition as an allied health profession with professional registration with the HCPC, creating a very narrow band of highly regulated professions. In contrast, the pluralistic Australian healthcare environment facilitates the development and self-regulation of new professions, as long as they achieve the requirements for self-regulating professions. The result is two very different allied health workforce profiles.

The limited sociological analysis on any of the allied health professions, let alone any cultural or political comparisons, limits our ability to explore these cultural differences within this book. It is, however, possible to briefly glimpse the impact of some aspects of culture on allied health practice, which highlights the way in which it has been constructed within, and built upon, largely Western values (Al Busaidy and Borthwick, 2012). For example, the theoretical basis of the practice of occupational therapy developed within a firmly Anglo–American background, reflecting the values and cultural norms of liberal democracies (Nettleton, 1997). Individual freedom and personal autonomy lie at the heart of liberal political ideology, in contrast to, for example, Middle Eastern monarchies or republics, which emphasise the 'collective identity' of family (Dwairy and Van Sickle, 1996).

For occupational therapists working in Arabic countries, there is a potential clash between Western care models centred on maintaining individual independence (client-centred goal-directed activity), and Arabic and Islamic paradigms focused on fatalism and family responsibilities (Awaad, 2003). In Oman, occupational therapy is a relatively recent import, initially established by professionals trained largely in the West. Al Busaidy and Borthwick (2012) found that occupational therapists had to adapt to Islamic culture, where it was more of a family responsibility to care for ill family members, and where dependence rather than independence was encouraged, with recovery viewed as determined by divine will (Yamey and Greenwood, 2004). In a similar vein, allied health professions may struggle in non-Western nations to match the freedoms to advance clinical practice in quite the same way (Tawiah et al, 2020). Tawiah et al (2020) found that there were several barriers to the development of advanced physiotherapy practice in Ghana, most notably, a powerful medical elite constraining allied health jurisdictions, alongside an absence in supportive legal frameworks to support it, and an absence of available postgraduate training opportunities to enable such change.

The training, distribution and employment of allied health in Asian nations appear to have a mixed history. For example, physiotherapists are well established in India (Rajan, 2014); however, a lack of documentation makes it difficult to determine the history of other professions in India or other Asian countries. Singapore and Vietnam have only relatively recently introduced in-country training for some allied health professions. China does not formally recognise allied health practitioners per se; however, there is growing evidence of the introduction of types of allied health services in China, such as the introduction of speech pathology and the delivery of physiotherapy-like training for existing health workers. In Chapter 2, the broader relevance of ethnicity in the allied health professions is addressed separately as part of an analysis of intersectionality in relation to diversity in allied health.

A further challenge for an international comparison of the allied health professions is the enormous variation in professional regulation in North America. For instance, in the US and Canada, allied health regulation is managed on a state-by-state level and varies by state, and there is no confederation of the allied health professions in either country. In North America alone, there are potentially dozens of variations in regulation and practice for each allied health profession. Consequently, we have contained the case studies in this book to an analysis of allied health in Australia and the UK, though we draw on some North American comparisons for illustrative purposes.

Allied health professions: migration and the global workforce

The international variations in perspectives on the allied health workforce impact on the global migration and uptake of the allied health professions in different countries. For example, while the nursing and medical professions enjoy a high degree of mutual recognition of professional qualifications, particularly across the European Union, the allied health professions generally do not.

In the UK, for example, international registration of allied health professionals by the HCPC is carried out on a case-by-case basis. The European Union's earlier 'sectoral directives' during the 1980s achieved a degree of harmonisation across some professions, such as nursing, medicine, dentistry and pharmacy, but it was a slow and laborious process (it took 13 years to agree a directive for architects) (Cuthbert, 2013). Competency standards were not uniform or easily comparable for all the professions, as was the case for the allied health professions, and a new mechanism needed to be found. Where automatic recognition was not possible because competency standards were not uniform, the European Union established a new system based on 'mutual recognition' instead of harmonisation. Thus, the European Union directive on the mutual recognition of professional qualifications (Directive 2005/36/EU, effective in 2005) enabled comparable baseline standards for recognition. However, standards across Europe varied, often considerably, among the allied health professions, and podiatry represents a case in point. Podiatry is a graduate profession in the UK requiring Bachelor of Science degrees awarded by universities in England and Wales (in Scotland, the degrees are four-year programmes); yet, in many other European countries, it is not a graduate profession. In some European countries, such as France or Germany, podiatrists complete two years of training (or less) outside the university or higher education sector. Consequently, freedom of establishment based on mutual recognition was, and remains, complex and difficult to solve (Editorial, 1999; Foo et al, 2016).

Equally, differing legal systems create difficulties when trying to establish common scopes of practice (Editorial, 2000; Foo et al, 2016). Indeed, podiatry is a good example more broadly as mutual recognition for podiatry is problematic even within Canada, where it is one of only a small number of health professions unable to agree on the mutual recognition of professional qualifications as part of the Agreement on Internal Trade (AIT), an aspect of the Inter Provincial Mobility Programme instituted by the federal government in 1995. The AIT was signed by the federal prime minister of Canada, alongside the premiers of the ten provinces and three territories. It was ultimately replaced with the Canadian Free Trade Agreement in 2017 to enable better alignment with freedom of movement and labour mobility across Canada, which states that where 'occupational standards for a regulated occupation are very different from one jurisdiction to another, a government may approve an exception to full labour mobility based on a legitimate objective' (see: www.workersmobility. ca/labour-mobility/exceptions/). One such legitimate objective is 'protection of human health', and podiatry is listed under 'exceptions by occupation', as are dental hygienists, medical radiation technologists, denturists, paramedics, nurse practitioners and midwives (see: www. workersmobility.ca/labour-mobility/exceptions/exceptions-by-occupation/). In effect, these provisions create obstacles to recognition even across provincial boundaries, which may or may not be realistically surmountable. For example, in the case of podiatry, the province of Alberta has established an exception on the grounds that as the scope of practice is so different in other provinces (Saskatchewan, Manitoba, Ontario and the North-West Territories are specified), 'these practitioners are not considered to be podiatrists' (see: www. workersmobility.ca/labour-mobility/exceptions/exceptions-by-occupation/).

Unlike Canada, there are no interstate restrictions to allied health practice in Australia due to the national regulatory framework, NRAS. Several allied health professions, including physiotherapy, speech pathology and podiatry, are recognised areas of skills shortage in Australia, which increases the opportunities for overseas trained workers to migrate to Australia if they meet a range of prescribed criteria for both professional registration and migration. In turn, migration is actively used to help manage areas of workforce shortage, though this has become increasingly contentious due to the inequitable burden on low-income countries, who often suffer net losses of health workers despite their greater need (Short et al, 2016). Eligibility to practise as an allied health professional in Australia is determined by the relevant professional registration board. The Physiotherapists' Board, for example, recognises the qualifications of graduates from specific universities in 19 different countries using a process called mutual recognition, which creates opportunities for streamlined eligibility to practise in Australia for people who also fulfil other migration requirements (Foo et al, 2016).

The Australian and UK health and social care contexts

The Australian and UK healthcare systems share many common roots, philosophies and principles. However, during the 20th century, both evolved in distinct ways that have influenced the direction and opportunities for the allied health workforce.

The areas of common ground stem from Australia's colonial origins. From 1828, English law was adopted as the law governing the early colonies of New South Wales and Van Diemen's Land. However, the colonies were given some licence to interpret and apply those laws according to local requirements. From a health regulation perspective, it appears that the colonies quickly adapted and adopted the regulatory systems being developed in the UK, in some cases, preceding the introduction of UK legislation. While the registration of medical practitioners and formation of the General Medical Council occurred in the UK in 1858, Tasmania and New South Wales had introduced legislation to regulate medical practitioners in 1837 and 1838, respectively. Victoria introduced medical regulation in 1862 (Carlton, 2017).

At the federation of Australia in 1901, the Australian constitution gave states the responsibility for the delivery of healthcare. For several decades, the Commonwealth had little input into healthcare (Hilless et al, 2001). The Commonwealth Department of Health was created in 1918 as a response to the need for a national coordination of health as a result of the Spanish influenza epidemic.

Healthcare was provided largely on a fee-for-service basis until the mid-20th century, with friendly societies providing access to some social benefits such as health insurance and unemployment benefits to members. A great deal of social and political reform occurred after the Second World War. The Commonwealth government introduced the Repatriation Commission for returned servicemen, resulting in an expanded role for the Commonwealth in health delivery.

A national proposal to introduce national health insurance in 1938 failed, as did several subsequent attempts over the following decade, including a proposal for free medicines. The Australian Medical Association (AMA), in particular, resisted free pharmaceuticals as an attempt to introduce 'socialised medicine'. The AMA successfully challenged the Commonwealth government in the High Court. Subsequently, the government held a referendum that resulted in changes to the Australian constitution. One of those amendments was the ability of the Commonwealth to introduce the Pharmaceutical Benefits Act 1950. Another effectively prevented any form of civil conscription, which ensured that medical practitioners remained self-employed and could not be made to provide medical services for a prescribed fee, nor could they be compelled to work for the government. This is a defining feature of medical practice within Australia and a key feature that distinguishes healthcare in Australia from the NHS (where general practitioners [GPs] became independent contractors) (Hilless et al, 2001).

In 1946, the Hospital Benefits Act gave control to the states to provide subsidised hospital care, ensuring free access for patients in public wards. This model of state administration of hospitals has continued, characterised by a mixture of public and private funding and delivery. Hospitals employ a range of allied health professionals.

A national health insurance scheme, 'Medibank', was first introduced in 1975, providing a government-funded reimbursement for a proportion of medical expenses. The scheme was modified by subsequent governments; however, since the late 1980s, Australia has had a universal, tax-funded health insurance system called Medicare. Medicare provides the whole population with subsidised access to the doctor of their choice for out-of-hospital care, free public hospital care and subsidised pharmaceuticals. There are also incentives for people to take out private health insurance, resulting in the current mixed system of public and private health funding.

Medicare provides some access to allied health funding for people with chronic illnesses (Cant and Foster, 2011). Various models are available but allied health services tend to be reimbursed on a fee-for-service basis (with some reimbursement from the state), require a referral from a GP and are restricted to a maximum number of appointments per year.

Another important and recent innovation of relevance to allied health was a significant shift in approach to and management of people with disabilities, from a medicalised (and largely institutionalised) model that gradually shifted in focus after the Second World War, to a social model that emerged in Australia in the 1980s (Butteriss, 2012). Of key importance was the introduction in 2013 of the NDIS, which is a national insurance scheme that provides support to people with disability, their families and their carers. The programme commenced in 2016 with a progressive national roll-out. The NDIS is jointly governed by the Commonwealth, state and territory governments, and replaces previous fragmented systems of disability support (Buckmaster and Clark, 2018).

An important component of the NDIS is the funding model. Instead of the previous model, which involved block grants to providers, effectively resulting in a geographic lottery for service users, the NDIS is an insurance-based scheme. Eligible service users are given funding packages determined by their level of need and self-defined goals. Ongoing funding for recipients is independent of time-limited contracts or annual appropriation cycles (Nevile et al, 2019). The NDIS is only available for people aged 65 years and under. People over the age of 65 receive care through the aged care system.

The NDIS is still relatively early in its implementation at the time of writing; however, evidence from pilot sites shows that the 'patient-centred fund-holding' model has significantly reorganised the way that disability services are introduced in Australia (Mavromaras et al, 2018). In particular, eligible participants have greater access to equipment services, allied health and integrated care. The NDIS workforce is still evolving. The area of greatest growth is likely to be in the disability support workforce but opportunities are also arising around service coordination roles, such as local area coordinators, and in areas of allied health (Wiesel et al, 2017). An allied health role that has emerged as a result of the reorientation of disability services is the DE, described in detail in Chapter 4.

In contrast to disability services, which have a maximum age limit, there is no minimum age limit for access to aged care services in Australia. Instead, access to aged care is determined on a needs basis. The aged care sector includes a wide range of services, ranging from those designed to keep people independent at home, to full-time, residential aged care facilities (including nursing homes). Support to keep older people independent at home is provided by the Commonwealth Aged Care Support Programme and, for higher-level needs, Home Care Packages (Australian Government, 2020). Packages of care are determined by a needs assessment, and include access to a wide range of health, social care, housing and home support care options. Services are means tested. Providers set the price for the services, and the government provides a subsidy for specific services based on the type of service and the ability of the senior to pay. Most older Australians (nearly 75 per cent) receive care at home or in community-based settings.

In many respects, the UK health system is more straightforward. The UK NHS was introduced after the Second World War and commenced operation on 5 July 1948. The NHS was proposed to Parliament in the 1942 Beveridge Report on social insurance and allied services.

The NHS was founded on the principles of universality and equity, designed to provide free care at the point of delivery, and paid for by taxpayer funding and national insurance contributions. The majority of healthcare in the UK is provided by the NHS; however, there is a small private component. According to the King's Fund (2014), approximately 11 per cent of the UK population hold private health insurance. The private healthcare market is diversifying in the UK, with increasing numbers of practitioners moving into the private sector or between sectors (Kings Fund, 2014).

Since its introduction, the NHS has undergone numerous political and organisational changes; however, the principles of universality have remained. In England, healthcare and policy are the responsibility of the central government, whereas each of the respective governments of Scotland, Wales and Northern Ireland is responsible for their own devolved models of healthcare. Each jurisdiction has responsibility for primary, secondary and tertiary care; however, the HCPC covers professional registration across all four jurisdictions.

The NHS is the major provider of healthcare in all four jurisdictions; however, the structure of each health service differs. One key feature that differentiates Australian and UK healthcare is that in primary care, GPs tend to work to a capitation model in the UK (in other words, they have a defined patient population). Other features of each of the four UK markets that vary in terms of their provision are the use of quasi-markets (contracting, commissioning, tendering and the use of individual budgets). With the growth of neo-liberalism, quasi-markets (particularly commissioning) have been a strong feature of the English healthcare system (Carey et al, 2020). Other features that vary between jurisdictions include: the extent of use of private providers; the cost of accessing social care; the use of performance targets; and the promotion of patient choice. Key to the differences between the UK and Australian healthcare systems are that, first, across all four jurisdictions in the UK, the government is still the largest central purchaser of services, even though they may purchase those services from different providers. Second, most of the health and social care provision is provided within the health and social care portfolios, whereas the portfolios are more fragmented in Australia. A third important distinction is the regional coordination of healthcare in the UK. The extent of centralised versus regionalised coordination of healthcare varies by nation, and has changed over time, but an important distinction between Australia and the UK is that healthcare in the UK tends to be regionally coordinated through service commissioning models.

Interestingly, in Australia, allied health professionals are employed across a wide range of sectors, including health, disability, aged care, education and justice. In the UK, the bureaucratic and ideological separation of 'health' from 'social care' has created much tighter distinctions around allied health roles and identity, where employees in 'social care' tend to strongly reject the 'health' label. For example, in Australia, social workers are recognised as an allied health profession by the AHPA, even though they may receive their training within a social science context. In the UK, social workers firmly identify as social care practitioners and are regulated separately to the HCPC.

A final important point for comparison is the training of allied health practitioners. In both Australia and the UK, most allied health practitioners are trained in state-funded universities. Some training is provided by a small number of private higher education providers. The UK has had a strong relationship over time between the NHS and education provision, with policy-level workforce planning tools guiding higher education provision for allied health providers. In Australia, in contrast, there is no central body responsible for workforce planning for the allied health professions. In the absence of workforce planning figures, higher education providers have largely been motivated by incentives that focus on increasing student numbers, rather than meeting specified population health needs. As a result, there has been a proliferation of new training programmes for allied health professionals in Australia over the past decade (McBride et al, 2018). In contrast, the removal of the provision of government grants for many allied health students in the UK has resulted in a substantial drop in demand for unfunded student places, and a concomitant decline in allied health training in the many allied health programmes in the UK (Beech et al, 2019).

The evolution of the allied health professions

The following section traces the key features that have shaped the modern allied health professions, and that will continue to shape it into the future. As we outline in detail in Chapter 3, several established allied health professions can trace their origins back to ancient therapies; however, their initial path to formal professionalisation occurred under (and because of) medical hegemony (Larkin, 1983) during the 19th century. As managerialism increased rapidly during the 20th century, so too did the decline of medical influence on the professional boundaries of allied health. At the start of the 21st century, allied health professional practice is largely determined by a managerial agenda, which emphasises patient safety and quality, with limited direct medical input into the scope of practice.

Turner's (1985, 1995) work emphasised the importance of medical dominance in shaping the structure and scope of the 'paramedical' professions, particularly in limiting their scope and authority to act independently. He stressed how medical influence within the regulatory frameworks of paramedical groups played a part in ensuring control and reserved a category of exclusion for those groups that were considered unorthodox, as reflected in their marginal position (such as chiropractic). However, the decline in medical dominance can perhaps be highlighted in a contemporary view of Turner's (1985, 1995) three versions of medical dominance. Subordination, where 'the nature and tasks of an occupation are delegated by doctors' (Turner, 1995, 138), no longer applies so clearly, if at all, as the allied health professions are no longer required to have medical representatives on their regulatory bodies. Exclusion (the fate of chiropractic in Turner's account, which could also include osteopathy) has shifted, with legislative recognition in place and more orthodox legitimation as members of the allied health group. But what of limitation? Certainly, professions like optometry and podiatry remain largely focused on eyes and feet, but the boundaries have blurred. It is no longer clear if the foot can be meaningfully isolated from the locomotor system of which it is a part, and the capacity to prescribe medicines may encompass new territories through the management of elements of systemic diseases that arguably impact on the foot. In each instance, the three modes of medical dominance, which once so clearly helped to differentiate the non-medical professions from medicine itself, are no longer quite so compelling.

While each allied health profession has had a unique inception and journey, we identify four phases that have been pertinent in shaping the allied health collective as we currently understand it, from a professional to a managerial framework. While the exact trajectory of each of the professions differs slightly and is influenced by jurisdiction, the global outcomes are largely similar, and have created a legacy for the evolution of the modern allied health professions. These are adapted from Larkin's (2002: 122) three phases:

1. The pre-professional phase
2. Medical registration
3. The formation of the medico-bureaucratic alliance
4. State control over healthcare

The 'pre-professions'

Wilensky's (1964: 142) 'Professionalisation of everyone' proposes that a starting point for all professions is 'to start doing full time the thing that needs doing'. Several established allied health professions have their roots in ancient therapies and techniques (Larkin, 1983). For example, early physical medicine techniques, including massage, manipulation, hydrotherapy and electrotherapy, had their origins in ancient civilisations and across multiple continents, including China and India, and later in Egypt, Greece and the Roman Empire (Nicholls, 2018). Later, during the 19th century, these therapies became organised under the disciplines of gymnastics, exercise therapy, bonesetting and massage.

The art of making spectacles and the understanding of optics also has ancient origins. Optometrists, or ophthalmic opticians, can trace the history of lens making and spectacle making to humankind's early understandings of the refractive properties of glass, nearly 8,000 years ago (Enoch, 2006). There is evidence of the organisation of the craftsmen involved in making spectacles at least as early as medieval times, and later through the Worshipful Company of Spectacle Makers (SMC), which was chartered in 1629 by King Charles I as an early form of protection and quality control of spectacle makers (Larkin, 1983).

While poorly documented, the history of podiatrists, or chiropodists, is traced to the 'corn-cutters', who were itinerant workers who provided their services on the streets and at fairs. Dagnall (1983) refers to ancient Egyptian footcare (around 2500BC) and the Ebers Papyrus of 1500BC, which described the use of olive oil and cow fat as treatments for corns. Dagnall (1983) proposed that an early text, entitled 'A treatise on corns, bunions, diseases of nails and the general management of the feet', by author Lewis Durlacher in the early 19th century secured the position of chiropody as a branch of medicine and surgery, and started the early ambitions for the professionalisation of chiropodists.

This notion of the 'pre-profession' is both a historical development and a normal evolutionary phase of most allied health professions. Most of the first allied health professions to achieve professional closure had long pre-professional histories (such as chiropody/podiatry and optometry), which involved clusters of skills and services that were later organised into formal guilds, and subsequently professions, largely following the Industrial Revolution and under the stewardship of medical hegemony. Millerson (1964) termed these groupings 'qualifying associations', which were seen as the precursor structures to formal professions.

Several new professions emerged during the 20th and 21st centuries in response to new technologies and changes in market demands. While these new professions lack a long pre-professional history, most have encountered a pre-professional phase that involves the provision of skills that have evolved to meet an identified need in the market, and the subsequent organisation and recognition of those skills into an identifiable profession. We explore these emerging occupations and their pathway to professionalisation in detail in Chapter 4.

The Industrial Revolution was a key turning point for the evolution of all modern professions, and indeed for the modern notion of the profession (Larson, 1977). Rapid advances in science during the 19th century, particularly in areas of mathematics, biology, physics and chemistry, led to the rapid growth of a new scientific basis for shaping and informing the healthcare professions. This also created technological breakthroughs that changed the way that healthcare was delivered. From a health perspective, some of the most significant of these included the discovery of X-rays, the principles of asepsis, a growing understanding of human anatomy, physiology and biochemistry, and the discovery and implementation of new forms of medications and anaesthesia. The same innovations, alongside improved public sanitation infrastructure and water, resulted in rapid improvements in public health (Szreter, 1999).

The development and rapid growth of organised manufacturing created new systems for defining and organising labour. The creation and commodification of labour markets meant that workers and work practices needed to be organised. In other words, pre-professions started to organise themselves into groups that would eventually become professions. The growth of manufacturing resulted in increased incomes for a growing proportion of the population, leading to the rapid development of the middle class. Access to increased leisure time created new opportunities to pursue and purchase new forms of health service.

From an allied health perspective, the Industrial Revolution created: an environment that stimulated demand for new services that could be consumed by the middle classes; new requirements for and systems of organising the workforce; and new technologies that enabled the rapid growth and evolution of some of the existing professions. However, the advances in manufacturing had a significant impact on several established occupations and their future development. For example, the mechanisation of lens manufacture in 1897 radically changed the economy and workforce of opticians from craftsmen who ground lenses to health practitioners with an interest and expertise in the prescription of eyeglasses.

The growth of industrial manufacturing also meant the end of some long-established craft guilds, such as shoemakers. In Chapter 4, we describe the professionalisation of the pedorthic profession (orthopaedic footwear manufacturing), which was derived from a long history of shoemakers that all but disappeared following the Industrial Revolution. Only small, niche workforces remained, one of which specialised in the manufacture and modification of shoes for medical purposes.

An important step in the formation of allied health professional identity was the development of training programmes. Various forms of early training programmes were developed from the late 19th century onward, such as certified massage training in Britain (Larkin, 1983). In Australia, early training courses for what were then massage therapists, the precursor courses to physiotherapists, were established by the AMA as early as 1906 (Chipchase et al, 2006), which later became physiotherapy training programmes. Early podiatry training programmes were established in London in the early 20th century but faced competition from army-trained 'foot orderlies'. The establishment of an accepted training programme was the first part on the journey to professionalisation for most allied health professions (indeed, all professions).

Training alone was not sufficient to prevent others from practising in evolving occupations' fields of work and the established occupational groups began to seek professional closure in the form of protection of their professional title. There were likely to be wide variations in practice standards and outcomes of work at a time when there was little scientific evidence to support any of the work of allied health practitioners (Larkin, 1983). The professional associations for many disciplines established early systems to standardise and accredit practice across multiple different providers and organisations. However, this did not prevent the untrained, or inappropriately trained, from using an otherwise unprotected title.

Medical registration

A key point in the history of all modern health professions was the registration of the medical profession (Larkin, 1983; Willis, 1989), which was pursued by the General Medical Council in the UK for some years before achieving success in 1858 (Berlant, 1975). Willis suggests that the period from 1840 to 1880 was the time that the medical professions in all Western countries attempted to secure statutory registration. In Australia, the former colony of Tasmania was the first to pass legislation to regulate medical practitioners in 1838, followed soon after by New South Wales (in 1838) and Victoria (in 1862) (Carlton, 2017).

While the medical profession, nursing and several allied health professions had existed in some form before this time, the regulation of medicine provided state endorsement for the medical profession, which united physicians, barber surgeons and apothecaries as a single professional group. This point cemented medical hegemony and the modern healthcare division of labour. It also created the structures that shaped the modern organisation and regulation of the health professions. As Larkin points out, the Medical Act 1858 did not provide the medical profession with an occupational monopoly, but it did provide a mechanism by which the medical profession was able to restrict access to public employment and various technologies by other craft groups.

Key features of these professional groups that brought them into contact with, and conflict with, the medical profession was, first, the timing of their professionalisation and, second, their competition with the medical model. Many allied health professions had long pre-professional histories. Therefore, the processes and drivers underpinning the professionalisation of the medical profession were also present for the early allied health professions.

The 'early professionalisers' had the same drivers for professionalisation as the medical profession as they sought to achieve professional recognition by the state and the public, as well as protection from encroachment by other occupational groups. Thus, their endeavours to clarify their own identity necessarily involved the codification of, and attempts to monopolise, unique areas of practice (Saks, 2016). However, the very codification of these practices under medical hegemony only made those tasks more visible to, and therefore prone to encroachment by, the medical profession, which was simultaneously attempting to clarify its own identity at a time when the science underpinning all healthcare practice was only just starting to gain traction as a defining feature of the professions (Larkin, 1983).

This era, until roughly the start of the First World War, was characterised by a lack of formal organisation of the health system. There was limited formal investment in healthcare, minimal intervention and control, and largely privately funded, fee-for-service healthcare. Medical dominance was a feature of a system in which state control was minimal and was important for shaping the repertoire of the allied health professions (Willis, 1989). The increasing organisation of the health system and managerial intervention by the state was replaced by a gradual, but concomitant, erosion of medical dominance within the health system.

Larkin (1983) describes the influence of the medical profession in defining (and restricting) the scope of practice of allied health professions in the UK over the past century due to its control over much of the legislation regarding health practice. As a large, organised and largely middle-class profession, the medical profession had access to status, resources and influence that were not available to the other emerging groups. The relationship between the patient and practitioner was key to accessing resources. Consequently, the emerging professions sought the patronage and support of the more dominant medical profession. Indeed, without this support, competing occupations (such as herbalists) faced enormous challenges in their goal for state recognition (Larkin, 1983).

Some nurses proposed that a nursing qualification should be a prerequisite for entry into the physiotherapy profession (Larkin, 1983), which would have resulted in physiotherapy being a specialist branch of nursing. However, nurses had not yet obtained registration and so were unable to formally adopt or endorse new clinical specialities. At the time, the focus was on preventing masseurs competing with the medical profession. The first attempts at registration involved voluntary registers of occupational groups that were supported by medical patrons.

It is logical to question why the allied health occupations were not subsumed as a sub-speciality based on their professionalisation alongside nursing and under the medical division of labour. The historic sequencing of the organisation and registration of the professions may have been pivotal in shaping the way that both nursing and allied health evolved over the 20th century. The separation of allied health from nursing is an important point that is revisited further in Chapter 7.

The medico-bureaucratic alliance

This period, which commenced approximately at the end of the First World War until the 1960s, has been described as a medico-bureaucratic alliance and signalled the growth of managerialism in healthcare. In the UK, the Ministry of Health formed in 1919, which marked the commencement of the involvement of the state in coordinating and financing healthcare (Larkin, 2002).

During this stage, the early health occupations sought to protect their professional titles and to emerge from medical dominance. While the medical profession did not directly control any of the allied health professions, indirect medical control was imposed by refusing requests for recognition by other occupation groups while tacitly supporting restrictive activities by the medical profession. Several examples of this tacit control are provided throughout the chapters in this book.

Several allied health professions attempted to seek separate state registration, including optometrists and chiropodists, but were blocked by the Ministry of Health because of perceived threats to the integrity of the medical profession. However, in response to the large number of 'medical auxiliaries' seeking registration, the BMA introduced the Board of Registration of Medical Auxiliaries in 1932. While this approach reinforced the subordination of the allied health professions, it was novel for its early introduction of a collective approach to the organisation of the allied health disciplines (Larkin, 2002).

In Australia, nine allied health professions achieved registration within every state and territory during this era (Carlton, 2017). There was strong evidence of medical dominance, as with their UK counterparts, but unlike the UK model, each profession was registered independently, not under a collective title.

State control over healthcare

The third stage involved a shift almost entirely to state management of the health professions. As Larkin (2002: 122) points out: 'In this last phase, the state is no longer the ally of one, but the regulator of all professions as it manages the now vast costs of health care.'

The timing and extent of state control varies between different jurisdictions. For instance, the formation of the NHS in 1948 was an explicit turning point for healthcare in the UK. The introduction of the Professions Supplementary to Medicine Act 1960 saw the registration of seven allied health professions overseen by profession-specific boards. Despite medical input to each of the boards, this was a strong shift from medico-bureaucratic control to state oversight of the allied health professions.

Generally, by around the middle of the 20th century, the state was taking an active interest in the regulation of both the health system and health practitioners. In Australia, healthcare was largely managed on a state-by-state basis, and the nationalised healthcare scheme came much later than the formation of the NHS.

However, what had evolved by the mid 20th century was a largely universal framework for the necessary minimum entry criteria for an occupation to be considered as a profession. These frameworks are reflected in most contemporary regulatory and licensing frameworks for the health professions (Health Care Professions Council, no date; Australian Health Ministers' Advisory Council, 2018), and dictate: the standards of entry (education and training); the mechanisms for maintaining those standards (the testing of member competence); the code of conduct; and the consequences for not adhering to those standards. These entry criteria are imposed in different ways for different professions, however.

The highest level of recognition is state regulation, which tends to include: legislative tools to enforce the standards; a register of practitioners who meet the standards; and, importantly, legislative protection of the title. In some jurisdictions, such as New Zealand, the US and Canada, professional scopes of practice are defined by law. This means that certain practices may be reserved for licensed professionals. For allied health professionals in Australia and the UK, this highest level of protection is largely historic, rather than risk-based, and both countries include state registration of professions such as podiatrists and occupational therapists.

The second level of recognition is self-regulation, in which the state grants permission to a third party, such as a professional body, to perform the tasks of regulation on its behalf. In Australia, the state has no way of intervening with self-registered professions. In the UK, professions that are self-regulated are overseen by the Professional Standards Authority for Health and Social Care, which accredits health practitioner regulatory bodies (state and self-registered organisations) and ensures they are adhering to appropriate standards of practice. Often, a self-regulating body enters into an agreement with a third party, such as the state or another funder, that recognises the endorsement of the self-accrediting body and provides additional benefits (such as payment) to the self-accrediting practitioners. This is known as co-regulation (Australian Health Ministers' Advisory Council, 2018). In Australia, this occurs with several self-regulated professions, such as speech pathology and dietetics, where their co-regulation gives them access to state (Medicare) funding for service provision.

A newer model called 'negative licensing' has recently been introduced within Australia. Negative licensing is an approach where there are no entry barriers to the practice of a profession, but individual practitioners can be prohibited from practising if they are found to be in breach of a regulatory regime, such as a code of conduct (Australian Health Ministers' Advisory Council, 2018).

It is becoming increasingly apparent that while the regulatory framework is predominantly designed to protect the public, not the professions, the application of the more controlled regulatory frameworks is largely historically and politically driven. The state regulation of some professions makes little sense from a public risk perspective. In Australia, for instance, the state regulation of occupational therapy makes little sense from a public safety perspective when compared with the co-regulation of speech and language therapy and dietetics.

Further, as outlined in numerous case studies in this book, several allied health professions are involved in the systematic deconstruction and reallocation of their core roles to other workers. This raises questions about the nature of regulated tasks and whether models of regulation need to consider the roles and functions of workers in isolation of their professional titles.

TWO

Diversity in the allied health professions

The allied health professions, and indeed all contemporary Western professions, have been shaped by a set of distinct social forces and contexts that were a product of their formative era. The Industrial Revolution saw the rapid organisation of labour at a time when social class, British colonialism and paternalism were dominant themes in much of the Western world. For the professions, the consequences have included a highly organised, hierarchical and strongly gender-differentiated workforce. Social policies have evolved over the past half-century to try to explicitly reduce gender and racial inequalities in education, the workplace and health service delivery, with varying levels of success in allied health.

This context is important for understanding both the evolution of the professions through a sociological lens, and also their contemporary context. In many ways, the world has moved on but the professions (particularly the highly structured and gendered health professions) are relics of their post-industrial era formation. At the start of the 21st century, the stereotypical allied health profession is still predominantly female, middle-class and white. The narrow analysis of any areas of diversity from an allied health perspective means that this is a limited field; however, there are dominant paradigms in the literature on the sociology of the professions that are important for diversity. Gender is the obvious position; however, ethnicity and socio-economic status are also important considerations.

Intersectionality recognises that social differences and divisions do not operate separately, but rather intersect. Examining diversity from an intersectional perspective enables us to consider that several classification systems coexist and interact – such as gender, ethnicity/race, sexuality, socio-economic status and even professional status – without reducing them to singular positions (Styhre and Eriksson-Zetterquist, 2008).

We found no analysis of the diversity of the allied health professions collectively, and only sparse discussion of the diversity within the individual professions. Yet, diversity, in all its forms, is important to understanding the social identity of the professions and how they came to their current position, their underlying assumptions about others and the world, and the way they are perceived by others. As with other chapters in this book, it is our goal not only to paint a picture of the current position of allied health, but also use this knowledge to help understand how the future can be shaped in a way that most effectively reflects the value of the professions to society.

Considering the allied health professions from an intersectional perspective, the literature focuses on three main areas, notably, gender, ethnicity and intra-professional hierarchies. Clearly, there is an interdependence between these three attributes but these issues, in turn, are examined through a range of different lenses.

Broadly, work addressing gender in the non-medical health professions appears to fall into three categories: historical accounts that trace the exclusion of women from, or subordination within, the health professions; contemporary re-evaluations exploring the feminisation of modern health professions; and works that establish the theoretical basis for examining gender within the health professions. Most focus on nursing, with a small number relating to professions such as pharmacy, dentistry, midwifery and physician assistants, and only a very few specifically related to allied health professions, such as physiotherapy, radiography or dental hygiene.

Interestingly, discussion of ethnicity has been almost invisible from the allied health profession discourse until relatively recently, where recognition of health inequalities has seen a growth in training in cultural competency, cultural safety and health literacy, alongside some attempts to increase diversity in student training.

As outlined in Chapter 1, the allied health workforce is itself a diverse mix of professions. This creates differences, divisions and stereotypes that have historically been shown to create power inequalities between the professions, privileging some and disadvantaging others. Perceptions of status differences between the professions influence their ability to attract students into the professions, for example, and also talk to the gendered issues within the allied health professions, not merely between allied health and medicine. This chapter also briefly explores the impact of interprofessional power relations in the context of gender and ethnicity.

Gender

The allied health workforce is highly feminised; however, it is not without variation. Several authors have suggested that the 21st-century gender divide in the professions is of the order of 70 per cent female to 30 per cent male, spanning countries such as Australia, the UK, the US,

Sweden and Norway (Hammond, 2009; Maclean and Rozier, 2009; Sudmann, 2009; Dahl-Michelsen and Leseth, 2011; Dahl-Michelsen, 2014; Nancarrow et al, 2017). The extent to which the allied health workforce is feminised has varied over time and across different nation states, as has the gender ratios between some of the professions within the broader allied health fold (Carpenter, 1977; Boniol et al, 2019).

Schofield's (2009) work confirms the extent of allied health feminisation in Australia, citing Australian workforce data to illustrate the point (76 per cent are women, excluding the radiography profession). A 2015 study from Victoria, Australia, of 27 allied health profession groups found that 83 per cent of the professions were predominantly female (Nancarrow et al, 2017). Again, however, there is some variation between allied health professions, with a number being highly feminised, such as speech pathology, occupational therapy, dietetics and orthoptics, and others far less so, such as chiropractic, osteopathy, orthotics/prosthetics and optometry. Interestingly, Schofield (2009: 387) commented on the Australian Health Workforce Advisory Committee (2006) report's conclusion that the losses to the allied health workforce were due to its 'relatively young and predominantly female' composition, implying that young, female staff would be likely to leave the service or become part-time in order to start a family, which she rejected as based on what she felt were assumptions rather than evidence, though this assumption formed the basis for a systematic bias against the entry of women into medicine at Tokyo Medical University. The proportion of women admitted to medicine dropped from 40 per cent to 18 per cent over a seven-year period due to the alteration of women's entry scores by the university, which admitted that it did not want to 'waste' medical education on women who would fall pregnant and leave the profession (Bishu et al, 2019).

The Victorian Department of Health and Human Services commissioned a large project into the allied health workforce (Nancarrow et al, 2017), the Victorian Allied Health Workforce Research Programme, which included an analysis of the gender breakdown of recognised allied health professional groups in Victoria. Figure 2.1 summarises these findings, which were derived from various data sources due to the lack of standardised data collection for allied health professionals, but indicate the relative gender breakdown of the respective professions.

In a comparison of 104 countries by the World Health Organization (WHO) (Boniol et al, 2019), women accounted for 67 per cent of

Figure 2.1: Percentage of women in allied health professions in Victoria

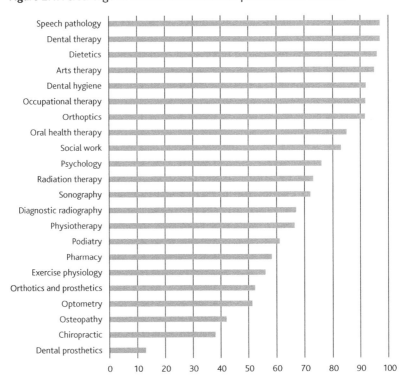

Sources: Victorian Public Sector Commission 2014, Australian Bureau of Statistics 2011, Australian Institute of Health and Welfare 2013, Professional associations 2015

workers in the health and social care sector but earned 11 per cent less than men when adjusted for working hours and occupation (28 per cent overall, unadjusted). In most countries, physicians, dentists and pharmacists are most likely to be male, though female participation is increasing in all of these fields and the workforce under the age of 40 is now more likely to be female. Female workers still comprise most of the nursing and midwifery workforce. The same study found that men are more likely to work in the private sector in highly paid occupations (for example, physicians) while women in lower-paid positions, such as personal care workers, were more likely to work in the private sector.

Macdonald's (1995) work is valuable in terms of both theory and social-political relevance in relation to patriarchy in the allied health professions. Macdonald provides a historical picture of the emergence of the professions at a time when modern industrial capitalism (or the market economy) was creating new forms of work, with far more differentiated tasks than had existed previously, in what was a complex division of labour. It was also a time that witnessed a 'rise of the rational scientific spirit', and these changes provided the impetus for the growth in professional occupations and their professional projects (Macdonald, 1995). The exclusion of women from the workplace can trace its origins to this point as the new division of labour largely comprised roles undertaken by men. However, as Macdonald points out, women held roles in pre-industrial society, based on folk knowledge (or 'status knowledge') rather than rational science but that nevertheless held value for society. The growth in scientific rationality during the industrial age also allowed the new, male-dominated health workforce to relegate or dismiss women's traditional knowledge as 'old wives' tales'. Macdonald (1995) cautions against the notion that there had been a previous golden age of women's emancipation from which they were torn as the new era dawned, arguing that institutional change, rather than capitalism per se, may have been equally responsible.

Witz's (1992) classic work on professions and patriarchy draws attention to the subordination of female professions within healthcare, focusing on medicine, radiography, nursing and midwifery. She provides a sociohistorical account in which the dominant male profession of medicine was able to constrain the roles of these professions through the exercise of social closure. Later, Macdonald (1995) crafted an insightful and penetrating account of the broader use of social closure as a means to establish and maintain patriarchal control within the professions generally, in both the caring and 'uncaring' professions.

Tracey Adams is a prolific author on North American professional feminisation and patriarchy in the non-medical, non-nursing health professions (Adams, 1998, 2003, 2004, 2005, 2010; Adams and Bourgeault, 2004). Using the example of dentistry to illustrate the patriarchal strategies of a male-dominated health profession, she identified the 19th-century ambition of dentists to be 'gentlemen' (Adams, 1998, 2010). This resonates with Macdonald's (1995: 124) remarks on the importance of respectability as a means to upward social mobility and to establishing a monopoly because those who had the means to consult professionals 'insisted on dealing with "gentlemen"'. For Adams (2010: 455), a 'gentleman' possessed what were regarded as essentially masculine characteristics: 'distinguished, rational, unemotional, authoritative, physically robust, committed to the job, highly educated and broad-minded … and scientific'; this effectively described a white, middle-class professional dentist. Women, conversely, were perceived as 'frail, emotional, dependent, less committed to employment; and somewhat narrow minded' (Adams, 2010: 455).

Adams identified several drivers for the feminisation of the health professions through the analysis of dentistry. These included: the introduction of equality legislation, reflecting changing societal values perhaps influenced by the feminist movement (Macdonald also highlights the passage of the UK Sex Disqualification (Removal) Act 1919 in reducing legal discrimination); increasing opportunities in higher education for women; and the impact of labour shortages and job growth on opportunities for women to enter the health professions, though Adams noted that both veterinary science and dentistry were feminising with no apparent labour shortage (Macdonald, 1995; Adams, 2010). Shifting social attitudes and better education are her favoured explanations here, along with one novel and important conclusion: immigration has played a part in feminising the health professions in North America. Adams cites the influx of immigrants from Eastern Europe, where health professions are more commonly female-dominated. Indeed, she points to the feminisation of medicine in both Portugal and the UK as being, in part, a consequence of immigration.

Witz's (1992) classic text on patriarchy also provides detailed explanations relevant to the feminisation of the allied health professions. Her analysis is illuminating in addressing not only the feminisation of radiography, but also the response of its own male members in attempting to destabilise it. Witz adds detail to Larkin's (1983) historical perspective and foundations in neo-Weberian theory by exploring the profession's own internal closure strategies – which Witz describes as internal demarcation strategies – in which the male members of the profession attempted to resist its rapid feminisation. For Witz, internal demarcation was exercised through discursive strategies that gendered certain roles and skills, and assigned a different value to them. The profession's male leaders stressed the importance of technical skills, which were associated with supposedly masculine traits, and diminished the patient-centred skills associated with female radiographers. As well as ensuring that the most senior and authoritative posts were reserved for men, these strategies also limited the feminisation of the profession and its apparently inevitable loss of professional status as a result. Unusually, in neo-Weberian terms, one key strategy of exclusion – the use of credentials (in the form of a diploma, introduced in 1921) – failed to act as a disincentive to female applicants, though Witz considers it to have been intended to do so.

Radiologists' demarcationary strategies aimed to distinguish between the technical acts of producing radiographs and the knowledge-based work of interpretation. This subordinated the role of the radiographer, who provided technically useful images to the physician to undertake the more complex work of reading the images and making a diagnosis. Although initially resistant to losing the right to report X-rays to physicians (having conceded the right to report directly to patients), the radiographers were outmanoeuvred by the radiologists upon whom they depended in the new division of labour around the medical use of X-rays. Without radiologists' support, the radiographers were unable to prevent the deskilling and loss of autonomy of those working in the private sector. It is here that Witz focuses on the gendered dimensions of change: the rapid feminisation of radiography occurring at the same time as the increasingly subordinated role of the radiographer. The subordination of radiography to radiology was accompanied by a more obviously gendered discourse in radiographer–radiologist relations (Witz, 1992). Witz holds the senior, male radiographers, in part, responsible for the subordination of the profession by acceding to the demands of radiologists, and, in doing so, setting in train the very processes that were to lead to its feminisation.

In 1936, a second attempt at exclusionary credentialism was enacted, lengthening training from one to two years, yet the numbers of female applicants continued to rise. Male radiographers then resorted to discursive strategies to limit feminisation, in which a revisionist view of the profession's history sought to portray the superiority of the engineering pedigree of radiographers, equating technical competence with masculinity and dismissing entirely the caring aspects as nursing.

What had been underestimated was the extent to which female nurses had prior experience of X-ray technology in the period shortly before the creation of radiography, and before regulation had been firmly established. X-ray nurses had been associated with early X-ray departments in hospitals, giving them an advantage when later seeking to gain access to radiography. Radiography training was hospital-based (not university-based) so prior experience was valuable and increased the likelihood of securing entry. Not only that, but the hospitals had been accustomed to employing nursing X-ray sisters to lead X-ray departments prior to the arrival of radiographers. This precedent favoured the employment of nurses with X-ray experience in managerial and senior posts as well.

Another flaw in the professionalisation of radiography was the failure of the professional body to pursue formal occupational closure via legislative means (Witz, 1992). Instead, the profession opted for 'medical patronage' in the hope that the power and influence of the medical profession might support its aims. Ultimately, employers reinforced gender segregation by favouring female workers with X-ray experience as they were cheaper to employ (equal pay between male and female radiographers was not sought by the professional body). For Witz, the subordination of radiography to medical dominance was accepted in favour of its submission to inclusion within the nursing profession, a more pressing danger for those who felt threatened by the authority and influence of the hospital X-ray sister and skilled X-ray nurses (Witz, 1992).

Conceptually, patriarchy has proven problematic and has suffered a lack of clarity, though the work of Witz (1992) has been instrumental in focusing attention on its prevalence and reproduction through the health professions. Macdonald (1995: 125, emphasis in the original) states that 'patriarchy is not merely *like* language; in one respect, it *is* language'. It is constituted not only in 'discursive strategies', but also in value-laden words that convey and perpetuate patriarchal beliefs. It is thus able to be reproduced at an almost unconscious level and needs to be actively addressed for our attention to be drawn to it.

Riska (2001) summarised the breadth of sociological approaches that might be applied to gender inequality, professional feminisation and gender segregation in medicine, which have clear relevance to allied health. Riska (2001) noted three main approaches: socialisation theory; neo-Weberian approaches; and the social-constructivist approach.

Socialisation theory, when applied to healthcare, relates to socialisation processes that shape gender traits and the development of 'sex roles'. Early socialisation, through the influence of family attitudes or school, may influence gender-related preferences for career choices, for example, or how female gender traits might limit professional advancement because of assumptions based on differing gender values. Equally, female gender traits may be an asset in circumstances where, for example, women may be considered advantaged in speciality fields such as paediatrics or elderly care because they may centre on emotional work at which women have been thought to excel (Riska, 2001). The feminisation of health professions may, in part, be explained by young women being offered more affirmative and achievement-focused role models as values change. However, Riska notes that the theory lacks explanations for the persistence of barriers erected previously, or changes in internal structures in a profession that might have resulted in new opportunities for women. Another version of socialisation theory might view the role of physician as gender-neutral given that they are all socialised in much the same way, stressing comparable values; however, to do so may render the gender-related issues invisible.

Neo-Weberian theory is based on the theory of social closure and explains the way in which power is exercised through exclusionary or demarcationary strategies, in this instance, in relation to gender. It remains the most potent theoretical approach (see the Introduction) but, for Riska (2001: 184), it has the disadvantage that it 'does not consider the impact of the changes in the status of [a given] profession on women's position within it and in this way makes gender invisible'.

The social-constructivist approach views health professions in terms of 'discourse', professions being viewed through the lens of gendered relations. It is here that discursive strategies are considered important in that they may be practised by dominant male professions.

Witz (1992) used both neo–Weberian and constructivist theories in her explanations of the control, subordination and feminisation of radiography. Riska considers that constructivist theory helps to focus on women's status within the health professions and grasps the importance of unravelling the social and cultural practices that define and establish the role of women in the division of labour. Its weakness is that it may be less able to consider the impact of the state on these processes.

Social closure, used to achieve exclusion and to pursue a professional project, is relevant to the exercise of patriarchy. Witz (1992) understood this and stressed the way in which (the less obvious) discursive strategies could be used to support other closure strategies, such as credentialing or legislative change. Witz expanded an existing framework of social closure theory, creating a matrix involving four main types of closure strategies adopted by male-dominated professions seeking to exclude, subordinate or marginalise women in the health division of labour. Each form of closure in the matrix involves strategies that explicitly (credentials, legislative change and so on) or implicitly (discursive gendered discourse) restrict female participation in a profession, or create boundaries between groups (either between or within professions) that disadvantage women.

Unsurprisingly, the professions most vulnerable to such strategies have been the 'caring professions', considering the way that the gendered discourse has valued the term 'caring'. Kennedy (2002) remarked on the contradiction inherent in the title. Abbott and Meerabeau (1998) drew attention to the way nursing acted to differentiate itself from the 'unqualified carer', that is, nurses are 'professional carers'. In making this claim, nurses exercise a version of occupational closure, establishing a boundary between them and informal carers or paid care workers who do not possess the required credentials. This implies that nurses have accepted as inevitable the mantle of carer; however, it is less clear if allied health professions would consider themselves in quite the same way.

Macdonald also raises the dilemma of trying to reconcile the requirements of professionalism with those of caring. For Macdonald

(1995), it is the 'expectation of objectivity' that is problematic. Professional judgement is based on a dispassionate weighing up of facts and knowledge, and should not be 'obscured by personal involvement or emotion'; yet, these very qualities are central to the notion of 'vocation' and 'dedication' that form part of the ethos of the caring professions. However, this has been used to characterise the course of nursing's professional project and its 'high risk strategy of using gender as the principal basis for closure', which, in stressing the qualities that only a women could bring, 'did facilitate the definition of an occupation that women could call their own' but effectively sealed its subordination (Macdonald, 1995: 154–5). Arguably, this is not the basis of the closure strategies adopted by the allied health professions, which have not attempted to emphasise their feminisation as a resource to support their professional projects. Rather, they have sought to minimise any emphasis on their increasing feminisation, while continuing to resist gender stereotyping and patriarchal discursive strategies.

Physician assistants in the US are an interesting example of a feminising profession, shifting from male dominance in 1977 to 60 per cent female in 2005 (Lindsay, 2005). The physician assistant is described as a 'dependent provider profession' that is essentially medical in nature. Lindsay found that the feminisation of the physician assistant role was not linked to deteriorating working conditions (the role was designed as a 'dependent provider' position in the first place), but associated with labour shortages in female physicians specialising in women's health and preventative care. However, the motives for joining were based on factors such as: a perception that the role was not broadly viewed as 'women's work' (unlike nursing); that it enjoyed high status as a form of medicine but involved less demanding work; and the fact that working fewer hours than physicians would not damage one's career opportunities, thus being viewed as amenable to family life. Lindsay also considers it possible that the development of feminist movements at the time that the profession began to feminise may have had a cultural role in suppressing active patriarchy. Like pharmacy, which experienced a rapid feminisation in the 1970s and 1980s, the physician assistant roles tend to be segregated, with men favouring self-employed positions and roles with greater autonomy (such as emergency care or surgical specialities) (Muzzin et al, 1994; Lindsay, 2005). Indeed, Lindsay (2005) links the loss of federal funding for speciality programmes for physician assistants as one possible reason for the decline in men joining the profession.

The gendered evolution of physiotherapy is interesting. As alluded to earlier (see Chapter 1), physiotherapy in the UK emerged as an essentially female profession in the 1880s, referred to as 'physiotherapist masseuses' during the Victorian era, at a time when prostitutes commonly used the title 'masseuse' in order to evade criminal proceedings (Nicholls and Cheek, 2006; Dahl-Michelsen, 2014). After such an inauspicious start, it was always likely to be an uphill struggle to effectively pursue a professional project. In order to distance itself from association with morally questionable behaviours, the nascent profession adopted strategies to desexualise its work on bodies, which involved preventing gender-mixed encounters between practitioner and client that would inevitably lead to 'ungovernable sensuality'; in short, it meant taking men out of the equation (Dahl-Michelsen, 2014: 674). Where males were to be treated, a (male) physician would be required to be present as a chaperone.

Yet, a different account of the profession emerges in Sweden, which developed earlier than in the UK (in 1813 according to Ottosson) and training was exclusive to men for 50 years (until 1864) (Ottosson, 2016). Indeed, it appears that the training programmes in Sweden at that time were effectively the sole source of physiotherapy education across the world, suggesting that varying sociopolitical and cultural factors altered the course of the profession in different nation states (Dahl-Michelsen, 2014). In Sweden, during the 1800s, the profession's exclusively male recruits were largely drawn from the military and those from socially privileged backgrounds, and tended to serve male clients. Although women were finally admitted in 1864, men still formed the majority by the turn of the 20th century.

In the first half of the 20th century, consistent with the ascendancy in medical dominance, conflict arose between physiotherapists and medically trained 'orthopaedists' over the training programmes. Although attempts to subordinate the physiotherapy profession included a plan to ensure only female entrants to training, which failed, the medical profession was successful in making the physiotherapy profession more subordinate than it had been previously (Dahl-Michelsen, 2014). After 1934, the battle was all but over as physiotherapy educational entry qualifications were lowered, and the training programme shortened in length, suggesting a highly significant deprofessionalisation and a reversing of the advances in its earlier professional project. In addition, it was developed as a female profession thereafter, and the preponderance of female physiotherapists within the profession continues to this day (Dahl-Michelsen, 2014).

Ottosson's (2016) work adds to the story of Sweden's physiotherapy development and juxtaposes it with the profession's development in England, adding insightful explanations for the shifting trajectories in each nation. Ottosson considered the early male-dominated physiotherapy profession in Sweden to have been 'displaced' due to a long drawn-out conflict between male physiotherapists and physicians in the latter part of the 19th century. Early 19th-century physiotherapy was a profession of high status and respect. It enjoyed good relations with physicians at the time given that the ascendency of medical hegemony had not yet been fully formed. It even established a physiotherapy assistant role, which was considered a female role. Ottosson (2016) examines why the shortened training time and lowering of entry requirements in the 1860s, which led to a rapid feminisation of the profession, was introduced without challenge. Male physiotherapists were preoccupied with waging an internecine struggle with physicians, who were entering a period of dominance and experiencing scientific advances that elevated their professional standing far above the physiotherapists. The battleground was over ownership of 'mechanical medicine'. As orthopaedics advanced more into surgical practice, aided by advances in anaesthesia, bacteriology and X-ray technology, their interest in physiotherapy techniques waned, and they began to regard the profession as a 'practical craftsmanship' with little place in the world of modern science (Ottosson, 2016).

The historical trajectory of physiotherapy in the US was somewhat different to that in Sweden. As an essentially female profession, it sought to avoid alignment with stereotypical views of women's work as caring and nurturing (Linker, 2005). However, it was still subject to the forces of exclusionary social closure by the dominant medical profession, and ultimately had to choose a form of subordination in exchange for recognition as a legitimate medical and scientific practice. Physiotherapy arose in the US during the First World War, when women were recruited (mainly from physical education colleges) to serve as physiotherapy rehabilitation aides in the rehabilitation of wounded soldiers returning injured from combat. In doing so, it rapidly assumed an ethos that emphasised the need for athleticism and physical robustness rather than the traits of nurturing, in part, because the therapy treatment was painful and so viewed as incompatible with nurturing (Linker, 2005). Indeed, it is interesting that Linker draws a clear distinction between the ethos of physiotherapy and that of nursing and occupational therapy, which much more clearly reflected Victorian ideals of womanhood. For Linker, not only was nursing still concerned with roles involving bedside nurturing, such as feeding and bathing, but occupational therapy emerged as a discipline designed to nurture anxious patients through the use of gentle forms of manual labour, including beadwork and woodworking (Linker, 2005).

Occupational therapy shared the same wartime influences and gender profile as physiotherapy but adopted a very different view of its role and contribution. Physiotherapists tended to work not at patients' bedsides (as did occupational therapists and nurses), but in gyms, engaging in physically demanding activities (Linker, 2005). By undertaking roles requiring physical strength as well as intellectual endeavour, physiotherapists sought to challenge the Victorian view that women were the weaker, more nurturing gender (Linker, 2005).

Gender is still relevant to the practice of contemporary physiotherapy and the potential for sexualisation where physical touching necessarily occurs in a more intimate form than in many other professions. Studies from the 1990s revealed that up to 70 per cent of physiotherapists and students, mainly female, reported experiences of sexual harassment from mainly male patients (McComas et al, 1993). Nicholls and his co-authors (Nicholls and Cheek, 2006; Nicholls and Gibson, 2010; Nicholls and Holmes, 2012) and Ottosson (2016) also offer sociohistorical accounts of physiotherapy and its relationship to the body, with clear gender relevance.

Dahl-Michelsen and Solbraekke (2014) explored the difficulties associated with learning clinical techniques during undergraduate training, where students are expected to practise on each other in a state of relative undress, which may involve mixed genders. They found that many of the desexualising behaviours employed during such encounters were initiated by females, who took greater measures than males to minimise sexualisation, such as the use of neutral 'sporty' underwear and avoiding that which might be construed as 'sexy'. Females also took more care in grooming, ensuring the removal of body hair from calves, legs and armpits, construed as part of a 'script' of femininity. Both male and female students expressed a preference for same-sex pairs when undertaking clinical skills training, which made the encounters easier to manage (which for females, included the absence of the 'male gaze'). Interestingly, Kennedy (2002) found that it was male students who experienced most discomfort with close physical contact and touching in mixed-gender practical work.

There is discussion of heteronormative masculinity in the context of male students working with other male students, and here a heterosexual script maintains the interaction. Overall, this was viewed as much less problematic than the potential for female–male sexualisation. Thus, physiotherapy, by virtue of the clinical skills and techniques that comprise its practices, is particularly exposed to sensitivities related to the treatment of bodies, and the potential for sexualisation, and thus serves as a useful exemplar of the importance of gender in the practice of the role itself (Dahl-Michelsen, 2014).

Adams's work examined the impact of gender and patriarchy in shaping the professions within the dental division of labour in Canada (Adams, 1998, 2004, 2010; Adams and Bourgeault, 2004). From the early 20th century, dentistry created a hierarchy by introducing a subordinate grade over which it had full authority: the dental assistant (Adams, 1998). Reflecting the attributes of their clientele, dental assistants were comprised of white, middle-class females. Their role was designed to reflect middle-class gender ideology, and comprised the combined function of 'a housekeeper, a nurse and a secretary/ book-keeper all at once' (Adams, 1998: 592). The dental hygienist was introduced after the Second World War to assist in providing preventative work, including tooth cleaning and advice. Unlike nursing, dental hygienists comprised a subordinate occupation uniquely designed for women by men (Adams, 2004). Training was provided by the Royal College of Dental Surgeons of Ontario, which also regulated the strictly supervised role. The professional project of dental hygienists was initiated in the early 1970s when the government transferred all allied health professions' education into a system of community colleges, thus reducing direct control over education by the dental profession. A further government review resulted in new legislation, the Regulated Health Professions Act 1991, through which dental hygienists, alongside many other allied health professions, achieved self-regulatory powers and the requirement to work under dental supervision was removed (Adams, 2004; Adams and Bourgeault, 2004). Hygienists were unable to practise 'licensed acts', including the scaling of teeth and some orthodontic work, without first obtaining an 'order' from the dentist, which meant that hygienists could not 'self-initiate' treatments.

For Adams and Bourgeault (2004), cultural feminism had been instrumental in achieving change as the professional leaders of the dental hygienists had recognised the political value of a feminist ideology, which supported their professional project. Indeed, feminist ideology underpinned their claim to government that they provided more accessible, 'egalitarian' services than dentistry by providing a more caring type of service, and argued that new legislation could counter gender inequality and expand consumer choice (Adams, 2004).

Choice of profession

Another important consideration in diversity is understanding individual preferences for specific professions. This is an area where intersectionality plays a large role. Gender, ethnicity and the nature of work are all interacting considerations in the choices that individuals make about their profession.

Kennedy (2002) explored the significance of gender socialisation in career choices and work perspectives for radiography and physiotherapy in the UK. Drawing on the contradictory notions of 'caring' and 'profession' (and professionalisation), Kennedy explored dichotomous identities common to both physiotherapy and radiography practitioners, who were torn between the values of a 'caring' profession (associated with female gender roles, such as domestic activities) and the ideas of a professional career more associated with male gender roles. The choice of profession was influenced by sociocultural and historical contexts, such as the influence of school and family for both males and females. For males, career choices were often based on prior experience of the professions; they did not initially consider the caring professions. Female entrants were more likely to select physiotherapy or radiography from a list of caring professions. Thus, earlier socialised ideas about gender-appropriate careers influenced their thinking. Males were less keen to work with sick, dependent people (in high-dependency wards, for example) as this demanded greater emotional closeness and caring, requiring skills that both male and female participants found more compatible with 'female nature', abilities, interest and identity. Although they perceived themselves to be gender-blind, many study participants revealed the importance of gender in their career decisions.

Kennedy (2002) found that male physiotherapists preferred to specialise in orthopaedic work and rehabilitation, while male radiographers distanced themselves from emotionally demanding or high-dependency work, or sought novel high-technology 'extended practice' roles. Radiographers more rapidly moved away from 'female specialities', retreating to higher ground as service managers, academics or researchers. Interestingly, female participants in both physiotherapy and radiography expressed no discomfort with high-dependency patients, accepted their subordinate role to the medical profession and continued to consider the 'caring' elements of professional work positively (Kennedy, 2002).

Later-career male radiographers were found to have been promoted quickly to senior managerial roles, whereas male physiotherapists tended to leave the NHS and move into private practice, enjoying better pay and higher status, reflecting the desire or perceived need to attain 'breadwinner' roles. These findings were reinforced in another, smaller study (Payne, 1998). In contrast, later-career female participants reported more varied roles and greater part-time work. Interestingly, females who had achieved higher-level managerial posts did not take any breaks in service (for example, maternity leave) and all worked full-time. Intriguingly, Kennedy (2002) concluded that most of the female participants accepted women's traditional gendered roles as wives and mothers, in spite of its detrimental effect on career advancement.

Dahl-Michelsen (2014) found that physiotherapy in Norway is subject to the same 'equality paradox', in that there is a strong tendency for labour market segregation – a significant point also noted in more recent popular scientific work addressing gender (Peterson, 2018). In particular, males demonstrate a preference for manual therapy and sports physiotherapy, whereas female physiotherapists appear to favour paediatric and psychomotor physiotherapy. Private sector work was also predominantly a male domain, with females working more often in the public sector.

Interprofessional diversity

Professional autonomy and the extent to which professions can exert relative influence upon the medical profession is an example of intersectionality, influenced by gender and interprofessional hierarchies. This is neatly illustrated in the travails of the profession of physiotherapy in Ontario, which was engaged from its post-war beginnings (as in the US) in a struggle for recognition within a male-dominated health hierarchy (Heap, 1995). Not only denied the right to make independent diagnoses by the dominant medical profession, it rapidly became embroiled in a jurisdictional dispute with chiropractic, a non-medical but male-dominated profession. Heap (1995) asserts that not only was the relative success of both the chiropractic and physiotherapy professional projects offset by concessions to the medical profession and the state, which prevented the acquisition of the full range of privileges and advantages sought by each, but the female-dominated profession of physiotherapy also suffered the greater disadvantage.

Although physiotherapy had in its favour a long-standing university education background, recruited from the middle classes and worked closely with the medical profession and in hospitals, it failed to secure insurance funding through the Ontario Health Insurance Plan (OHIP). Chiropractic, an essentially primary care-based profession, did not require a physician's referral and could set up in private practice and obtain fee-for-service remuneration via OHIP. Chiropractors could also use and interpret X-rays, a significant authorised act. By 1991, when the legislation for regulated health professions was introduced, and cost became a key consideration, the Canadian Physiotherapy Association sought to argue that chiropractic was too expensive, dangerous in its use of full-body X-rays and lacked a legitimate scientific background. Ultimately, it failed to dislodge chiropractic from its position within the field, and Heap (1995) implies that the feminisation of physiotherapy may have played a part.

A similar trajectory was faced by physiotherapists in the US. After the war, physiotherapy rehabilitation aides adopted the title of 'physiotherapist', formed a professional body and focused on a professional project aimed at securing a place in the division of labour as a scientifically credible and educated workforce. The new American Physiotherapy Association (APA) quickly distinguished itself from nursing by pointing out that its courses were of four years' duration (as opposed to the three years in nurse education), in addition to which they had wartime training as manual therapists (Linker, 2005). However, without the secure employment provided during wartime, the nascent profession entered the competitive world of the private sector, where osteopaths, chiropractors and nurses all claimed physiotherapeutic expertise. The medical speciality of electrotherapeutic physicians also laid claim to the title, and demanded that it be exclusive to male medical graduates (Linker, 2005). If that were not enough, it also insisted that the APA be renamed the American Physiotherapy 'Technician' Association, ostensibly to avoid public confusion but, in reality, to establish a subordinate grade of practice through 'demarcationary' closure (Witz, 1992; Linker, 2005).

The Great Depression unfolded at a time when most people paid for medical services themselves, health insurance was limited and managed care was inchoate; therefore, competition for scant resources forced the APA to concede ground in exchange for formal recognition by medicine. In doing so, the APA sought to ensure that physiotherapy was acknowledged as integral to the medical establishment. The price to pay was a loss of any claim to make a diagnosis or to determine treatments, which would in future be overseen by physicians, though the right to independent private practice was retained (Linker, 2005).

Implicit within the discussion of gender is the gendered nature of roles and work. The nature of work roles is tied up with professional status. As the aforementioned examples have illustrated, masculine work is associated with a dispassionate objectivity, that is, with technical, scientific roles that might be construed as 'uncaring' (Witz, 1992; Macdonald, 1995; Payne, 1998; Kennedy, 2002). Males exhibit a preference for manual therapy and sports in physiotherapy rehabilitation and orthopaedics (Kennedy, 2002; Dahl-Michelsen, 2014), athleticism and robustness, gymnastics (Linker, 2005), and gentlemanly pursuits (Adams, 2003). Men are more likely to choose autonomous roles and to be self-employed (Lindsay, 2005). In contrast, the aforementioned studies have painted female roles as caring, dependent, working with sick people, emotionally demanding (Kennedy, 2002), acting as a housekeeper, nurse and secretary (Adams, 1998), and preferring roles that are family-friendly and compatible with a family lifestyle (Lindsay, 2005).

It is no surprise that there is a strong interaction between high-status roles and those that are deemed more masculine. In an analysis of professional status within the podiatry profession, the following tasks were identified as being associated with higher status (Borthwick et al, 2009): more specialised, sports-related tasks (as with physiotherapy, a background in human movement was valued); more medical tasks, including surgery and an ability to order X-rays; and providing expert advice rather than hands-on technical treatment. Status was influenced by public perceptions of the profession, which was, in part, influenced by public awareness that university training was required to become a podiatrist. The employment setting only influenced status according to the level of responsibility or skills of the specific role, though there was recognition that pay could be higher in the private sector.

In examining the roles with high levels of feminisation (noting that these demonstrate international variations), the consistently more masculine professions are osteopathy, chiropractic, diagnostic imaging medical practitioners, radiation oncology medical physicists and diagnostic imaging medical physicists (Nancarrow et al, 2017). These roles all fit the criteria for both perceived status and more masculine tasks that are more technical and scientific, as well as more sport or biomechanically oriented.

Ethnicity

Of all the areas of sociological analysis of the allied health professions, ethnicity is one of the least well explored. Like gender, social attitudes to ethnicity have altered radically over the past few centuries, with different issues and considerations facing different national jurisdictions. The emergence of the allied health professions over the past century, and within a Western orthodox medical model, has shaped their perspective and interactions with society. The tendency of the Western orthodox medical model to be a normative framework has shaped the interactions of allied health with 'other' (non-white, non-Western) populations (Abreu and Peloquin, 2004). Reflecting this normative frame, the discussions of ethnicity within the allied health professions tend to come from two perspectives. The first perspective reflects a desire to reduce health inequalities and explores the challenges faced by the allied health professions in meeting the needs of diverse populations in terms of racial, cultural and socio-economic needs. This literature examines issues around equity of access to services, as well as cultural competence, health literacy and cultural safety. The second perspective is the issue of workforce diversity, which is largely explored through a lens of inclusion and assimilation – in other words, ensuring equity of access to under-represented groups in the professional training and delivery of allied health professions.

Reinforcing the white, middle-class origins of the professions, Black (2002) provides an insight into the historical development of the profession of occupational therapy and its practitioners' origins in the US during the 1900–20 period, characterised as comprising essentially single, white, highly educated, middle- or upper-class young women. Indeed, it was only in 1943 that consideration was given to admitting anyone other than white middle- or upper-class women into training. At the same time, it was decided that 'coloured' people should be eligible to train as occupational therapists; however, in an era of segregation, separate training at 'coloured institutions' was required (Black, 2002). By 1985, minority black and ethnic groups comprised 8 per cent of the occupational therapy workforce in the US, leading to new recruiting programmes seeking more men and black, Asian and minority ethnic (BAME) students.

The concept of health inequalities is well documented (Cena et al, 2002; Sobo et al, 2020), and it is not within the scope of this book to explore these issues epidemiologically. The disproportionate burden of illness was brought into firm focus during the global COVID-19 pandemic, which revealed striking evidence of the higher incidences of morbidity and mortality among minority black and minority ethnic (BME) groups in the US (Price-Haywood et al, 2020) and the UK (Cook et al, 2020), exacerbated by poor access to healthcare. These same issues are relevant in terms of equitable access to allied health services (Hill-Briggs et al, 2010).

Cena et al (2002), writing on occupational therapy, observed a lack of acknowledgement of ethnicity in occupational therapists' clinical writing, which, it was argued, rendered visible the minority ethnic group as 'other', while failing to remark on the status of the 'norm'. This is an idea derived from the notion of 'marked' and 'unmarked' cases from within linguistic anthropology, such as, for example, a female paediatrician or a male occupational therapist (Evans, 1992). Within the guidelines on clinical documentation adopted by the American Occupational Therapy Association, cultural and socio-economic history was only considered relevant where it might indicate prior levels of support (Cena et al, 2002).

Cena (2002: 131) suggest that this absence of discussion signals that the 'silence and evasion of discourse about race' also exists in the broader 'health and rehabilitation discourse', which prevents the professions from establishing equality in service provision. For Cena et al, the predominantly middle-class and white European-American make-up of occupational therapy defines sociocultural norms, which are reflected through bias in professional practices. Interestingly, Cena et al (2002: 131) suggest that the reluctance of European-American health professionals to acknowledge race and thus racial inequalities may stem from a 'graceful, even generous liberal gesture' by avoiding the issue (see also Morrison, 1994). However, in so doing, it effectively 'denies reality' through ensuring the absence of race.

Cultural competence is an approach that has been used increasingly by the allied health professions to help address inequalities in healthcare delivery awareness of, and sensitivity to, cultural issues through knowledge development and self-reflection (Pitama et al, 2018; Gray et al, 2020). Cultural safety takes this concept further, to include an understanding of the sociopolitical issues that may manifest as power imbalances and racism (Gray et al, 2020).

Several professions have developed approaches to introducing cultural competence with a view to reducing health disparities (Brusin, 2012; Abrishami, 2018; Maldonado and Huda, 2018). One study, reported by Yeowell (2013a), suggested that some services view minority ethnic allied health practitioners as the 'experts' in cultural competence, leading to the assignment of patients from BME backgrounds to those practitioners from a similar background.

Radiography undergraduate programmes seek to embed cultural competence from the start, ranging from service user questions during the admissions interview, through to service user-led sessions involving storytelling (of personal experiences of radiography), service user feedback in practice and interprofessional conferences (one-day events) addressing cultural competence (Harvey-Lloyd and Strudwick, 2018).

An Australian study makes the case for a broad cultural competence education and training across the allied health professions, which aligns both diversity within the healthcare patient population with the values of tolerance and understanding necessary to the success of interprofessional working and harmony (Hamilton, 2011). In aligning the difficulties of 'profession-centrism' with 'ethnocentrism', notably, cultural and linguistic misunderstandings and stereotyping, addressing the two broad issues collectively is viewed as a key advantage (Hamilton, 2011).

A number of studies acknowledge the importance of language and the challenges of communicating sometimes complex instructions to multilingual patient groups (Shams-Avari, 2005). Yet, taking steps to enhance access to competent translation services does not solve the problems of cultural competence, as illustrated in a number of striking case examples where, for example, professionals may mistakenly report parents for child abuse as a result of failing to understand cultural practices with which they are unfamiliar (Shams-Avari, 2005).

Chau (2020) makes the point that cultural diversity poses particularly complex problems for radiographers, who must attempt to communicate effectively in short encounters involving technical requirements in often stressful circumstances for patients and resulting in potential risks for patients if they are unable to follow instructions (Chau, 2020). Similar issues of language in radiography have been identified in other countries, notably, multilingual countries such as Ghana (Antwi et al, 2014) and South Africa (Wyrley-Birch, 2006). Chau (2020) cites a number of studies reporting underuse of health services by minority ethnic groups in Australia, New Zealand, the US and Canada, including concerns about undergoing diagnostic imaging examinations. These may be related not to language difficulties alone, but to cultural differences and a sense of being stereotyped in some way. Echoing Cena et al (2002) and Hammond et al (2019) in relation to occupational therapy and physiotherapy, respectively, Chau (2020) reports the fear of making mistakes or seeming to appear discriminatory among some educators and practitioners in radiography. For Chau (2020), cultural competence is more than mere knowledge; it is an investment in trying to connect with those who are different.

Australian optometrists sought to advance cultural competence and engagement with minority ethnic groups in a more meaningful bid to improve health service use and outcomes (Truong and Selig, 2017). Truong and Selig (2017) point out that more than 26 per cent of the population was born overseas, and that 67 per cent of new arrivals, alongside 49 per cent of longer-standing immigrants, speak a language other than English at home. Optometrists felt that they had no formal model or framework guiding or assisting their approaches to eye care with minority ethnic groups (Truong and Fuscaldo, 2012). Truong and Fuscaldo (2012) found that practitioners described eye health beliefs among other cultures as 'old wives' tales', whereas those with culturally homogeneous practices were more inclined to assign differing beliefs to a lack of education, age or socio-economic background. In addition, having to adjust practices to ensure greater spatial distance from female patients was evident when dealing with Muslim patients (Truong and Fuscaldo, 2012). Recommendations for the optometry profession included: the adoption of a national cultural competence framework; the development of policies of priority of access for disadvantaged groups; and engagement with local cultural groups to better understand their eye care needs (Truong and Selig, 2017).

Cultural competence among dental health professionals has been explored in a variety of environments, including Australia and New Zealand (Nicholson et al, 2016), as well as Mumbai in India, where the vast majority of respondents claimed to provide culturally competent oral health provision yet nearly half struggled to define what it meant (Savant et al, 2016). Health literacy is another common concept adopted by health professionals in the context of accessing and supporting diverse populations. Health literacy refers to the ability of individuals to access, understand and use health information (Brooks et al, 2020). As with cultural competence and cultural safety, the concept of health literacy is still not widely understood or consistently applied by allied health professionals (Brooks et al, 2020).

What is abundantly clear from the literature across the allied health professions is that allied health outcomes and access to services for minority ethnic groups remain problematic, despite efforts to enhance cultural competence in education programmes. Wider societal factors undoubtedly play a role, such as socio-economic status, as well as cultural perspectives, particularly in the recruitment of minority ethnic students to allied health programmes. It is equally clear that there remains a dearth of literature on ethnic diversity and cultural competence in the allied health professions, which are, in turn, viewed as essentially white, middle-class and mainly female occupations. Work may need to be done to enhance awareness of cultural diversity within the allied health professions, as well as measures put in place to better inform and promote them as viable, attractive career options for all.

The under-representation of minority ethnic groups in allied health training programmes has been a long-recognised challenge in the UK, US, Canada and Australia, in part, because of the disproportionate burden of illness on those groups (MacDonald and Rowe, 1995; Greenwood and Bithell, 2005; Grumbach and Mendoza, 2008; Donini-Lenhoff and Brotherton, 2010; Komaric et al, 2012; Moore, 2018). There is limited literature on the reasons for the poor rates of uptake, and few published systematic approaches to addressing them. Inadequacies in cultural competence had already been exposed in a study in which physiotherapists struggled to provide services to the Bangladeshi community, reportedly due to language differences and a lack of cultural awareness (Jaggi and Bithell, 1995). For Greenwood and Bithell (2005), this was a problem spanning all the allied health professions across the UK, which had failed to represent the population they were treating.

A 1995 UK study exploring reasons for the poor recruitment of minority ethnic students to occupational therapy programmes highlighted the need for revised admission processes, curricula and ethos to improve minority ethnic recruitment (MacDonald and Rowe, 1995). A survey of secondary school students identified low rates of intention to study allied health by BME groups, and that admission grades were a barrier to entry (Stapleford and Todd, 1998). Physiotherapy has also struggled to address the issue of race, ethnicity and cultural competence in terms of recruitment to the profession (Mason and Sparkes, 2002). In 2001, only 5 per cent of physiotherapy students were drawn from minority ethnic groups in the UK (the latter constituting 8 per cent of the UK population), though this improved to 10 per cent by 2011 (Yeowell, 2013a) and approximately 19 per cent of student admissions in 2017/18 (Hammond et al, 2019).

Approaches used by speech and language therapist programme admissions teams in the UK aimed to enhance applications through measures such as: positive images in recruitment literature (featuring minority ethnic students); liaising with local schools, colleges and bilingual teams; overseas recruitment fairs and university outreach schemes; and providing articles and publications in minority languages. However, most courses reported a distinct lack of success in achieving better minority ethnic recruitment as a result (Stapleford and Todd, 1998).

Cultural influences have been found to impact on allied health as a career choice. Two studies reported that some Asian students regarded physiotherapy not as a profession at all, but as an occupation of relatively low status. Physiotherapists were thought of as essentially 'masseurs' and thus, by implication, somewhat uneducated (Greenwood and Bithell, 2005; Yeowell, 2013b). Greenwood and Bithell (2005) also reported that minority ethnic respondents were less likely than white respondents to be aware that physiotherapy and nursing were degree-level programmes. Black Caribbean respondents more often considered physiotherapy to be a 'woman's job', and thus unacceptable for males. Indeed, family responses to career choices were identified as more important for minority ethnic students, with physiotherapy being perceived either as a 'woman's job' or, in the case of Muslim students, a profession in which female students should not treat male patients (Greenwood and Bithell, 2005).

Similar findings about the perceived lower status of the allied health professions have been reported in speech and language therapy, which struggled even more than physiotherapy to recruit effectively from minority ethnic social groups (Stapleford and Todd, 1998). Indeed, Stapleford and Todd (1998) discovered that most minority ethnic applicants to allied health courses (physiotherapy, dietetics and speech and language therapy in this study) were Indian and black Caribbean candidates, with very few Chinese or Bangladeshi students. Applications to allied health programmes were relatively few in contrast to the high numbers of applications of certain minority ethnic school leavers to well-known and prestigious programmes, such as medicine or law (Stapleford and Todd, 1998). Interestingly, a survey of physiotherapy students compared the occupational status of physiotherapy in Australia and England (Turner, 2001), and found that physiotherapy is considered to be a higher-status profession in Australia than in England. The high status of physiotherapy in Australia is reflected in the high demand for university training courses.

A later study by Greenwood et al (2006) also adopted a questionnaire tool to explore attitudes to speech and language therapy with school and college students in the process of considering university courses. It was already known that recruitment to the profession had a deep gender divide, with very few males choosing to study speech and language therapy (Boyd and Hewlett, 2001). The results showed poor levels of awareness of speech and language therapy as a profession, lack of awareness that it required degree-level training, and that it was perceived as unscientific (Greenwood et al, 2006). Students from a BME background listed the wishes of the family, studying for a degree, a high-status job and good remuneration as important considerations, whereas white students were concerned more with working in teams and meeting people. Some respondents suggested that those from minority ethnic groups may speak with an accent that would not be either suitable or acceptable within speech and language therapy (Greenwood et al, 2006).

The aspects of touch, gender and undressing constituted a deal-breaker in terms of family and community acceptability (Yeowell, 2013b). Similarly, Pakistani female patients expressed discomfort at receiving treatment from male physiotherapists, or engaging in mixed-sex group exercise programmes, leading to low compliance and attendance rates (Yeowell, 2010).

For Hammond et al (2019), the sense of 'otherness' is a recurring feature, based on the 'default physiotherapy student identity' as white, middle-class, mature and female. Indeed, for Hammond et al (2019), class and socio-economic background intersect with ethnic background, emphasising difference and alienation. Cultural differences add to the mix, where some Asian students felt that their reserved demeanour was at odds with the default identity in terms of the model outgoing, gregarious and confident physiotherapist, while, conversely, black students were reluctant to adopt such a manner for fear of being more easily construed as aggressive or rude (Hammond et al, 2019). What was perhaps original in this work was the reported 'micro-aggressions' of the white staff, who may have been entirely unconscious of their transgressions, or were trying to avoid highlighting race or ethnicity, and, in doing so, amplified them. Examples ranged from differing expectations of academic outcomes, touching and avoiding eye contact with BAME students (Hammond et al, 2019). Students also became adept at modifying their manner to more closely fit the 'default identity', such as in speech, which meant emphasising a clear diction in the manner of the middle classes (Hammond et al, 2019). For Hammond et al, this study provided a unique insight into 'unmoderated student perspectives', and thus afforded the audience access to an honest and perhaps deeper level of BAME experience.

Despite the multicultural population of Australia, diversity of access to allied health training has received scant attention at a policy level. The discussion that does exist largely focuses on the inequalities with the Aboriginal and Torres Strait Islander populations, and strategies to both increase the representation of the indigenous workforce within allied health and increase the use of Aboriginal and Torres Strait Islander health practitioners (Lai et al, 2018; Wright et al, 2019). Rather than a process of assimilation, as is largely used by other allied health professionals, Aboriginal and Torres Strait Islander health practitioners are primary care practitioners for whom evidence of identity or acceptance of being an Aboriginal and/or Torres Strait Islander person are one of the criteria for registration. They work alongside existing health practitioners and sometimes autonomously in the delivery of culturally competent care to Aboriginal and Torres Strait Islander communities.

Conclusion

This chapter has explored the complex interplay of the intersectionality in the allied health professions. Gender and the patriarchal origins of the health professions have shaped professional repertoires, the roles individuals adopt within their professions and their interrelationships with other professional groups. The picture is far from complete and requires further investigation, but clearly the allied health professions need to understand the way their gendered histories can influence their current and future opportunities.

The role of ethnicity, cultural competence and cultural safety is poorly understood within the allied health professions. All professions face challenges of how to best meet the needs of culturally and linguistically diverse populations who may also experience other inequities that impact on their health and wellbeing. The heterogeneity of the allied health professions mean that each discipline will face unique challenges in best meeting the needs of their specific populations and in a variety of contexts.

THREE

The established allied health professions

The largest recognised group of allied health professionals is comprised of the established state- and self-regulated professions. These professions have claimed clear philosophies and sometimes anatomical domains and scopes of practice that differentiate them from each other, and other emerging disciplines. This chapter draws on the examples of optometry and radiography, one of which was established prior to the advent of the era of medical dominance, and the other during it. It thus illustrates the way allied health professions responded to the challenge posed by medicine in defining the new health division of labour that took hold in the early 20th century. It also illustrates the different ways in which these professions later identified with other allied health professions: one as part of the broader collective; the other remaining separate from it (Larkin, 1983; Boyce, 2001, 2006). As was explained in Chapter 2, and should be borne in mind when considering the context of the account that follows, they also serve as useful exemplars of the contrasting gender divide within the allied health professions. Radiography became a primarily female profession, and optometry remained a mainly male profession (though, interestingly, the former remains stable but the latter is becoming more feminised) (Register, 2010; Healy et al, 2015).

Those allied health professions with a long pre-modern history – that is, the groups that emerged prior to the period in which medical dominance became firmly established – experienced medical opposition and resistance in their bid for recognition and state registration during the early to mid-20th century (Larkin, 1981, 1983, 2002). Equally, those that emerged during the period of ascendancy in medical authority experienced the same forces at work. Thus, the neo-Weberian framework is key to understanding the development of these professions, and its various strands become immediately clear as the story unfolds, both the strategies of exclusion, limitation and subordination of the medical profession, and the resistance of the allied health exemplars as they attempted to advance their own professional projects (Saks, 2015, 2017, 2018). As medical hegemony became firmly established, a 'medico-bureaucratic alliance' emerged, allowing medicine to assume both social and cultural authority in determining healthcare priorities on behalf of the state (Larkin, 1983). As a result, the medical profession began to enjoy an unprecedented influence over the health division of labour, and thus to exert control over other, non-medical, health professions (Saks, 1995). In this chapter, then, the theory that best explains the unfolding drama is drawn from the neo-Weberian perspective, which highlights the strategies of social closure (medicine's attempts to exclude, and optometrists and radiographers attempts to usurp) and professional autonomy (as the allied health professions struggled to defend their own boundaries) within a context of growing medical dominance. The medical profession adopted three identifiable 'modes of domination', applied to the different allied health professions, illustrating the potency of the neo-Weberian perspective (Turner, 1985, 1995).

These three variants (outlined in the Introduction) neatly capture the distinct fields of some of the allied health professions, while simultaneously drawing them together as part of a single, dominated collective. In response, each of these professions attempted to mount some form of resistance. In some instances, this meant attempting to form bridges and alliances with other allied health professions, but in other cases, it led to a calculated separation from other groups. Each mode of control exerted by the medical profession reflected both the strengths and the particular weaknesses of the professions subject to each variant. For example, those professions that claimed expertise in treating disorders of a specific body part were more easily contained and exposed to limitation within a narrowly defined field of practice. Optometrists, dentists and podiatrists (specialising in eyes, mouths with teeth and feet, respectively) fell into this category (Turner, 1985, 1995).

Those that already worked interdependently with medicine, such as in hospitals, were subordinated to medicine and compelled to work under medical direction. Nursing, midwifery and radiography constituted exemplars of this mode of control. Finally, professions that were underpinned by heterodox paradigms that did not align with the ascendant biomedical models of mainstream medicine were more easily excluded. Unorthodox practices were considered unscientific and consigned to the margins of legitimate healthcare. Osteopathy, chiropractic and homeopathy were thus excluded from the legitimate scientific healthcare community. Furthermore, their refusal to submit to medical control cut them adrift from mainstream healthcare provision. For Turner (1985, 1995), their marginal status was confirmed by the absence of regulatory or legislative recognition (though this changed later, during the early 1990s, for osteopathy and chiropractic) or their inclusion in the UK's NHS.

Nevertheless, the three variant forms of medical dominance continue to serve as useful ways to explain the different routes undertaken by the allied health professions as they emerged and developed within the penumbra of medical power. They also allow us to address the variation in trajectory of key exemplars from within the broad field of allied health, which further illustrates the tensions between attempts to retain autonomous, independent practice while, in some cases, adopting a defence based on collective resistance (Boyce, 2006).

Why did some allied health professions seek shelter and advancement through alliances with broadly comparable groups, while others opted to remain separate and fight for recognition independently? Indeed, was it always a matter of choice? For example, some of the older, more established professions, whose history pre-dated the growth of modern medicine and the modern health services, followed different paths in this regard. Optometrists and podiatrists both trace their historical forms back at least to the 17th century. Both focus their claims to expertise on a particular body part (eyes or feet). Each was established within the private sector (prior to the state provision of healthcare) and was thus linked to both the provision of healthcare and commercial business. Both were small compared to medicine and established a number of professional bodies that adopted differing viewpoints on how to negotiate with medicine. Yet, ultimately, in the face of 20th-century medical dominance, one (podiatry) sought refuge within the allied health collective as a 'profession supplementary to medicine', while the other (optometry) favoured the opposite course of action.

Unlike radiography or physiotherapy, each practised independently of medicine, working autonomously and separately, without direct contact with, and thus dependence upon, medicine. Radiography, by contrast, emerged later, being established firmly within the hospital sector and thus working intimately with and alongside medicine. It started in a co-dependent position with medicine, without autonomous practice beyond the daily reach of medicine. As the cultural and social authority of medicine grew, it was more easily able to establish and maintain control over optometry through the stratagem of limitation, and over radiography through direct subordination. A closer examination of these two professions provides some of the answers to the questions posed earlier, and illustrates the conundrum faced by each in navigating a way through medical hegemony while attempting to secure professional status, recognition and independence.

Optometry: allied to medicine or allied to itself? A case of splendid isolation

The case of optometry serves as a particularly good example of the professionalisation of a non-medical health occupation with a long 'pre-modern' history, and how this has influenced its subsequent trajectory. In part, this was facilitated by the way in which its practice was confined to one body part and, within that, to a clearly defined (and restricted) scope of practice. It was initially able to establish a foothold in the health division of labour before medical dominance became fully established, as did podiatry and, to some extent, physiotherapy. The case of optometry is interesting as it is a health profession that continues to be associated with commercial gain and retail business, in apparent contradiction to the altruistic orientation assigned to professions in the early professionalisation literature (Barber, 1963). On that basis, it is difficult to sustain a 'functionalist' perspective of the profession given that the value of professions to society supposedly stems from an ethical and altruistic form of service, not one motivated by financial gain. Rather, it is the neo-Weberian perspective that affords a clearer insight into its story. Optometry was able to navigate an independent course through the 20th century, finally acquiring separate state registration without being classified as a 'profession supplementary to medicine' in the UK. In some ways, it was the first 'test case' of the success of medical imperialism as its increasing threat to medical authority was contained through limitations to both scope of practice and claims to diagnostic skill, enshrined in legislation, in both the UK and Australia (Cole, 2015b). Today, optometry retains its status as an independent profession, and is not considered to be part of the 'allied health' fold in the UK (unlike Australia, where it is). Yet, its recent development has aligned closely with other allied health professions, most notably, in its acquisition of independent prescriber status (Needle et al, 2007). Indeed, as we shall see, the dilemma facing the profession in respect of the prescribing of medicines is paralleled in both the UK and Australia.

In the UK, optometry developed independently of the collective group of professions 'supplementary to medicine', partly because of its established position in the marketplace as an autonomous group, but primarily because, unlike many other allied health professions, it claimed to have a scientific knowledge independent of medicine (Larkin, 1981). As an occupation founded on scientific principles, where its practice largely developed independently of medicine, this claim offered a unique defence of its stature and its right to independence. In contrast, podiatry, similar in so many respects, did not enjoy any such claim. On the contrary, podiatry claimed to constitute a legitimate branch of medicine and surgery (Dagnall, 1995a, 1995b, 1995c). The Royal Charter granted by Charles I to the SMC in 1629 established early recognition for the specialist skills and scientific knowledge of practitioners. Further advances in knowledge of optics and optical science followed in the 17th and 18th centuries (including the work of Isaac Newton), and the ophthalmoscope and ophthalmometer were invented in 1851 and 1853, respectively (Larkin, 1981, 1983). A decade later, Frans Donders, attributed as the founder of optometry, published the first path-breaking text on the treatment of optical defects of accommodation and the scientific use of refraction (Larkin, 1983).

By the early 20th century, the British Optical Association (a competitor organisation to the SMC) claimed that these advances were made by physicists who were, in effect, early optometrists, despite the fact that some were medically qualified. At the same time, medical interest in optics and the specialist field of ophthalmology was marginal throughout the 19th century. This was to change in 1906 with the first attempt at securing an Act of Parliament establishing the rights and recognition of optometry. Undermined by both internal conflict between competing optometrist organisations and the power of the medical profession, the Bill failed. However, the scene was set for an ongoing jurisdictional dispute and a battle for the recognition of optometry as a legitimate, independent, autonomous profession that did not reach a conclusion until state registration was established in 1958 (Larkin, 1981, 1983).

Increasing state involvement in healthcare during the early 20th century played a crucial role in alerting the government to the debate, which tended to side with the medical profession given that the cultural authority of medicine was largely accepted. A second bid for chartered status by the British Optical Association in 1919 failed due to medical opposition, and in the interwar years, the National Health Insurance scheme led to the insurance companies favouring the cheaper costs of using optometrists instead of medical ophthalmologists. However, the latter concern was sidestepped by the assurances given by the BMA that GPs would not charge money for initial sight tests, and a Royal Commission sided with the medical authorities, which encouraged recognition of 'dispensing opticians' instead, who would, in effect, be technicians working under medical direction (Larkin, 1983). However, the aim of state registration was considered possible at some point, and the new Joint Council of Opticians (an amalgamation of previously competing optometry bodies) pursued it further. Nevertheless, the

BMA feared that state registration would enable optometrists to become 'eye doctors' and vociferously opposed it (Larkin, 1981, 1983). Initially, the first apparent concession was to recognise optometrists employed in medically controlled clinics by the Ministry of Health, though this suggested an effective subordination by removing any right to independent practice. However, a lack of sufficient numbers of doctors prompted the recognition of 'opticians' under the terms of the National Insurance Act 1936, enabling them a limited form of state acknowledgement, granting those with the requisite diploma exclusive access to insured patients (Larkin, 1981, 1983).

At the inception of the NHS in 1948, the government faced an even greater expansion in demand for eye services, providing another opportunity for optometrists to make a case for registration. On the other hand, it presented medicine with an opportunity to subordinate optometry through incorporation into expanded medical services under medical supervision (Larkin, 1981, 1983). However, the optometrists were in an advantageous position because the service could not run without them – and they knew it. In confronting medical opposition, they outlined medicine's economic concerns and its lack of interest in what was best for the public. By refusing outright to join the proposed new eye clinics (which would place them in a subordinate position to medicine while losing the right to independent practice in the private sector), they threatened to derail the government's plan for enhanced healthcare provision in eye care. With such leverage at its disposal, the now-unified optometry profession pushed for legislation and registration on more favourable grounds. Although initially concerned to avoid alienating the medical profession by stalling on progress, the government recognised that a solution would need to be found to enable the sort of healthcare promised in its pledges on healthcare. Finally, it agreed that a General Optical Council should be created, and three registers established (one for opticians testing sight and dispensing glasses; one for those testing sight only; and one for the 'dispensing opticians') (Larkin, 1983). Title was to be protected but scope limited and any claims to making a diagnosis excluded. The medical profession was successful in ensuring firm representation on the General Optical Council and the requirement that opticians refer any 'suspected' cases of eye disease to ophthalmologists. The Optician's Act 1958 both established the independence of optometry and simultaneously limited its scope of practice and curtailed any future ambitions through statutory control.

Both optometry and medicine gained some success after conceding ground, and it was in the interests of the government, acting as the final arbiter, to agree a compromise between the two given its reliance on both to deliver on its new health service agenda. Thus, optometry was able to achieve state registration with protection of title and exclusive control of the market in sight tests and spectacles, yet did so without having to depend upon the broader support of the collective group of allied health professions that shortly thereafter became the professions 'supplementary to medicine'. Indeed, it achieved just as much as the latter, without losing its distinctive, individual identity or separate control over entry and training. Nor was it entirely subject to terms of registration that would leave it as a vassal profession, merely 'supplementary' to the overarching control of the medical profession. However, it was somewhere in between: it retained its identity and separate status but remained subject to the influence of medical dominance, just as the other allied health professions had been. It lost any right to the treatment of eye disease (other than the correction of accommodation defects with spectacles) or any right to make independent diagnoses.

A not dissimilar picture emerged in Australia, though the timings differed. What dogged the educational development of Australian optometry was the dispute with medicine over scope of practice, just as it had been in the UK. It had been limited to a narrowly defined role, largely refractionism, and only assumed some responsibility for early eye disease detection much later (as was the case in the UK). Indeed, Willis (1989) considered the treatment of eye disease to be relatively uncontentious but the detection of eye disease as central to the dispute between optometrists and ophthalmologists. No one disputed the right of optometrists to dispense and sell spectacles, and no one disputed the right of ophthalmologists to treat eye disease by surgical or medical means; it was the territory in between that led to a major jurisdictional dispute between the two professions (Willis, 1989). Indeed, Willis (1989: 130) makes the point that optometry differed from the other professions subject to 'limitation' by medicine essentially because, unlike pharmacy or dentistry, it was faced by a medical speciality that directly competed for the same occupational jurisdiction in the form of ophthalmology. It was less a dispute between optometry and medicine, and more a conflict at the boundaries separating optometry from ophthalmology. The development in the 19th century of the British ophthalmic optician and dispensing optician provided the later basis for the Australian differentiation between optometrists and optical dispensers. Early development of ophthalmology in Australia paralleled that in the UK, with early pioneers developing the field in the 1860s, culminating in the establishment of a recognised speciality through the creation of the Ophthalmological Society in 1899, only 19 years after the UK equivalent (Willis, 1989). However, the emergence of optometry in Australia followed some time later, details of which are scant.

Indeed, Willis (1989) offers an explanation for the relative absence of data, asserting that historical accounts tend to be written selectively, primarily addressing the interests of the middle and upper class, whereas the working class, from which opticians originated, receives very little attention. The creation of the Victorian Optical Association in 1911 marked the beginning of the professional project of optometry in Australia, when plans for educational and legislative closure were first laid out. It quickly began to distance itself from its 'trade' origins, adopting a professionalising ideology which aped that of dentistry and medicine (Willis, 1989). Divided between its two key functions at the time – testing vision and selling spectacles (the former a professional activity; the latter commercial in nature) – the professional ideology of optometry began to develop, drawing the profession ever closer to conflict with ophthalmology. In 1918, the Australian Optometrical Association was formed, and by 1921, it had issued a code of conduct recommending a voluntary limitation of scope of practice in order to avoid provoking the medical profession – an interesting facet of medical dominance to which Willis (1989) draws our attention. Where the Australian profession began to differ from its UK counterpart was the attempt in 1919, by the Victorian Optical Association, to change the title from 'optician' to 'optometrist' in a bid to clearly separate itself from the optical dispensers. By then, ophthalmologists had disputed the right of optometrists to test for visual defects (but not to dispense spectacles) on the grounds that it required the use of drugs, and only medical doctors had access to such medicines. By straying into the territory of ophthalmology, the optometrists had sparked a conflict over scope of practice. An attempt to secure the registration of 'sight-testing opticians', drafted in 1913, failed to materialise after being roundly criticised by the Ophthalmological Society. Registration was achieved, however, in Tasmania (in 1913), Queensland (in 1917), South Australia (in 1920) and New South Wales (in 1930), lending weight to another bid by the Victorian profession. However, for Willis, the failure to subordinate optometrists meant that ophthalmologists were forced to limit their practice. Having failed to stop optometrists undertaking sight testing, they sought to ensure that no one would be registered with exclusive rights to do so, thus enabling the ophthalmologists to continue to charge a fee for sight testing as well.

It appears it was the support of the large and influential commercial wholesale optical companies that helped to enable the Victorian Registration Act 1935 as they too felt threatened by ophthalmologists' plans to exclude optometry from the market. The Act did not restrict sight testing by non-registrants, but did restrict the use of the titles 'optician' and 'optometrist'. Optometry was limited by statute to sight testing and spectacle provision, with no access to drugs and no right to test for eye disease – a very similar picture to that in the UK. Established as the Australian College of Optometrists in 1940, the Victorian professional body decided, by 1960, to adopt a new title – one it was better able to justify given that its reach did not extend beyond the state boundaries of Victoria (Cole, 2015a). As the 'Victorian College of Optometry', it could more easily access state funding and avoid accusations that it was 'pretentious' in claiming national leadership when it was essentially a Victorian organisation. Optometry in Victoria had already secured state legislative recognition in 1935, via the Opticians Registration Act, giving the registration board full authority to determine education and training standards. Prior to the Act, education was largely piecemeal, comprising part-time, three-year professional fellowship courses or even correspondence courses available in the US. In fact, the majority had acquired the necessary skills through apprenticeships or were self-taught (Cole, 2015a). The registration board set about its professional project by establishing a committee to devise a new curriculum that would model itself upon the profession in the US, where four-year university education programmes were the norm. Its revised entry criteria were equivalent to university entrance requirements, and, remarkably, were uncontested by the committee's two ophthalmologists – the medical representatives that had gained seats on the board in 1935. The Act itself had been bitterly disputed by Victorian ophthalmologists, who claimed it would 'license ignorance and quackery' (Cole, 2015a: 412). Even the University of Melbourne, empowered under the terms of the Act to veto the programme, declined to approve a four-year programme, suggesting that it would 'encourage opticians to give opinions on and treat disease' (Cole, 2015a: 412). However, the programme's advocates on the registration board persisted and finally agreed a compromise in which a four-year programme would be approved in return for a prohibition on optometrists 'giving medical or surgical treatment' (Cole, 2015a: 412). Cole (2015a) suggests that this was a strategic error on the part of the university as it had no authority to determine any such prohibition on treatments, which remained a matter for government alone. Having agreed to proceed, the first course eventually began in 1941, culminating in a Diploma of Licentiate of Optometric Science. Although not quite a degree, it nevertheless established a four-year university programme that was not matched in any other state for another 20 years.

With the dominance of the medical profession fully established (Willis, 1989), it was not until 1961 that a degree programme was finally achieved and delivered, eventually becoming a Bachelor of Optometry degree in 1994. Although both optometry and ophthalmology were excluded from government financial support in the National Health Act of 1952 (ophthalmology thus being the only medical speciality unable to access health insurance benefits), ophthalmologists found ways to circumvent the Act and secured an advantage through private health insurance funds, enabling them to recover 75 per cent of fees (Willis, 1989). In 1975, access to the new national health insurance programme, 'Medibank', was granted to optometry.

In the 1960s, the college finally attained a degree programme, though it had already incorporated modern techniques into the curriculum, such as fundus lens examination, binocular indirect ophthalmoscopy or scleral indentation (Cole, 2015a). In Victoria, limited access to a number of drugs began in the 1960s, and access to prescription-only medicines was secured in 1996, mirroring a shift to independent prescriber status being recommended in the Crown Report in the UK in 1999 (Cole, 2015a).

Optometry: allied to itself or allied to others?

More recently, there is evidence to suggest that modern optometry has tended to be swept into the broader 'allied health' division of labour when seeking certain advantages, in common with other similar groups. It continues to defend its independence and singular identity, and has largely survived changes in market conditions and the growing neo-liberal policies of recent decades without being depleted or diminished by them. Yet, its professionalising ambitions have meant that it has sought to expand its scope of practice, knowledge and skill range.

One key exemplar of its efforts to advance its authority, market power and professional prestige is to be found in its attempts to secure independent rights to prescribe medicines, particularly those classified under the UK Medicines Act 1968 as 'prescription-only' medicines. Like podiatry, its scope of practice was curtailed by its exclusion from the terms of the Medicines Act 1968, which recognised only doctors, dentists and veterinary practitioners as eligible to access prescription-only medicines (those medicines deemed to constitute such a risk to public safety as to demand limited, specialist rights to prescribe them).

In this respect, its trajectory mirrors that of the podiatry, midwifery, nursing and paramedic professions in its bid to recover lost ground following the Medicines Act 1968, and its attempts to expand and extend into new task domains underpinned with new knowledge and expertise. Boyce's (2006) thesis that the allied health professions had adopted a distinct 'profession community' was intended to reflect the changes in the allied health professions since 1980, and her construct was developed from work undertaken in the 1990s. It does not imply a loss of professional identity within each of the constituent groups, only that workforce demand and a shifting policy agenda forced those groups to work together to achieve common political and professional goals (Boyce, 2006). Thus, it is fair to apply the notion of 'professions allied to each other' within that context, and to view the development as a step beyond the 'professions supplementary to medicine' achieved in the 1960 Act, which registered many as professions for the first time.

Central to the thesis of the 'profession community' was the context of neo–liberalism, enhanced competition within health service provision and state reluctance to further the cause of professional monopolies, which were increasingly viewed as anachronistic, self-serving and an obstacle to workforce flexibility. Ageing populations, fewer available younger workers and increasing technological specialisation represented new pressures on the health service workforce and those state authorities required to maintain viable, safe and effective care (Nancarrow and Borthwick, 2005). In such a climate, workforce flexibility became a prerequisite to achieving a sustainable healthcare provision, in which there was no place for professional monopolies. As a result, new organisational structures emerged that encouraged the development of organisational as well as professional identities, as cogently reported in Carmel's (2006) work on the allegiances of different professionals in a specific organisational speciality, such as intensive care.

Allied health developed as an alliance designed to give a voice to the smaller professions (non-medical, non-nursing) at the policy level, which earlier organisational structures did not allow or actively encourage. For Boyce (2006), the final stage in the development of the subculture of the 'profession community' was the 'institutional phase', in which extra-organisational allied health associations acting on behalf of the collective group would emerge, encouraging and facilitating a growth in collective identity. In the UK, this is clearly evident in the formation of the Allied Health Professions Federation, which acted to initiate policy changes on the rights of a number of its constituent professions to prescribe medicines. In this context, optometry prescribing is viewed as evidence of its continuing separation from the allied health fold as it did not need to rely upon the collective lobbying strength of the federation to further its own claims to prescribing status. It was, however, subject to the same processes and prejudices, notably, medical dominance and state uncertainty as to its credibility as a safe and effective option. It also had to undergo the same scrutiny as the other allied health professions, requiring ministerial approval to proceed with a submission, and needing to persuade the Commission on Human Medicines (CHM) of the appropriateness of its case. It was, therefore, very much in line with the other professions seeking similar status, and its progress towards independent prescribing bears this out.

The restrictive terms of the Opticians' Act 1958 were foregrounded when the profession sought to expand its access to medicines as part of its professional growth and advancement. As it increasingly sought to treat a wider range of eye problems than it had previously, it found that the Act had limited the profession's ability to do so. Consequently, many of the medicines it sought to treat these minor eye conditions were unavailable to it as the Opticians' Act had prevented opticians' treatment of conditions of the eye beyond those related to accommodation – in other words, sight testing and the provision of spectacles (Titcomb and Lawrenson, 2006; Borthwick, 2008). Equally, it was limited to identifying 'suspected' eye diseases, without the right to make independent diagnoses, though it had been accustomed to using medicines that were used in the diagnostic process. The result was an occasional but piecemeal series of amendments to medicines regulations to allow optometrists access to a few additional medicines, either to aid the diagnostic process or to treat minor conditions; however, these were cleverly curtailed by the specification that many such medicines were for administration only, rather than supply to patients. This denied optometrists the ability to supply medicines to treat minor conditions within their scope of expertise, thus limiting them to one-off treatments as part of a single patient consultation (Borthwick, 2008). As health policy began to change in the late 1980s, reflecting the ascendancy in neo-liberal ideology and the impending marketisation of health services, opposition to restrictive practices grew, particularly where they were viewed as obstacles to the modernisation of service provision (Exworthy and Halford, 1999).

The advent of managerialism, its use of 'purchaser–provider' systems of competition and tendering for contracts, combined with a growing realisation of the demographic changes occurring in Western nations globally meant that changes to restrictive regulations limiting flexibility and responsiveness were more likely (Flynn, 1999). In 1989, a consolidated Optician's Act was established, removing some of the restrictions evident in the original 1958 Act (Needle et al, 2007). Following the consolidated 1989 Act, in 2000, the UK General Optical Council was able to amend the requirement that 'suspected' eye disease must be referred to a medical doctor, affording greater autonomy and authority to optometrists in practice. At more or less the same time, the 1999 Crown Report review of the prescribing of medicines concluded that professions other than medicine and dentistry should be eligible to become prescribers, and identified optometry as an early candidate for 'independent prescribing' (Department of Health, 1999).

Shortly thereafter, in 2005, very significant advances were enabled by new legislation recognising optometrists as 'supplementary prescribers' of medicines (Titcomb and Lawrenson, 2006; Borthwick, 2008). At the same time, further exemptions to access, supply and administration rights of prescription-only medicines were enabled for 'additional supply' optometrists (who had undergone extended training), as was full access to 'pharmacy-only' medicines, finally giving optometrists freedom to treat a range of common, non-sight-threatening eye disorders, such as infective and allergic conjunctivitis, blepharitis, and 'dry eye' (Titcomb and Lawrenson, 2006; Borthwick, 2008). The General Optical Council had carefully put in place a programme of education, training and regulation to prepare for 'supplementary prescribing' status, and found, to its surprise, relatively little opposition from the Royal College of Ophthalmologists (Rumney, 2019). Clearly, the next step would be to recognise optometrists as independent prescribers, and this duly followed, with enabling legislation in place by 2008 (Rumney, 2019). Independent prescriber optometrists are registered with the General Optical Council on a 'speciality register', identifying them as holding additional qualifications/skills above the threshold level of registration, similar to the use of 'annotations' by the HCPC for allied health professionals (Rumney, 2019).

Where they differ is that optometrists must register their defined scope of prescribing practice and reregister every year, separately to their 'normal' registration, for which they must also declare their current prescribing practice (Rumney, 2019). This means that should an optometrist change role, and enter a management or an academic role, they must declare it, which may, in turn, have implications for their ongoing speciality registration. All of this reflects the extent to which optometry sits outside the allied health fold and forges its own path in terms of education and regulation.

Curiously, there are similarities with other allied health prescribers in terms of demographics, with about 5 per cent of the optometry profession qualified as independent prescribers (there were 14,500 optometrists in 2018), and relatively few in Wales or Northern Ireland, with those in England mainly working in the new 'Hospital Eye Service'. In Scotland, 20 per cent of community optometrists work to a new NHS contract – the remainder do not have access to NHS prescribing funds. It is also worth noting that in optometry, independent prescribing is a postgraduate qualification only in the UK; it is an accepted part of the undergraduate programmes in the US, Australia, Canada and New Zealand (Rumney, 2019). This remains the case even when the UK has a lower per capita number of ophthalmologists than any of these other countries; the UK College of Optometry is reluctant to change, unlike nursing and pharmacy in the UK, where plans for 'prescriber-ready' undergraduate programmes are being considered (Merrifield, 2018).

Optometry prescribing in Australia has met with more consistent opposition from the medical profession, though it varies between states. Victorian legislation enabled access to a broad list of prescription-only medicines in the mid-1990s while restrictions continued to apply to the profession in the Australian Capital Territory (ACT) and New South Wales, with Queensland lagging even further behind. In the latter case, although legislation was gazetted, strenuous objections by ophthalmologists led to threats to walk out of the public health system – to effectively go on strike – thus delaying implementation by several years (ACT Health, 2007). Indeed, the AMA opposed a bid by optometrists to secure funding under the Pharmaceutical Benefits Scheme (PBS), describing optometrists as 'medical pretenders' (Borthwick et al, 2010). Even by 2012, the AMA was vociferously opposed to optometric prescribing outside 'strict co-management plans', in itself a reluctant compromise to the demands of Health Workforce Australia to enable greater non-medical prescribing (Hambleton, 2012).

The restrictions on optometry prescribing in the UK may reflect an excess of caution by the General Optical Council when drawing up the standards it felt would be necessary to persuade the medical profession to agree to them. In doing so, it disadvantaged itself in relation to other allied health professions, which did not adopt such restrictive standards. It is likely that this happened because optometry forged ahead of the allied health groups in achieving independent prescribing first, independently of others, just as pharmacy and nursing did. It is also probable that the allied health professions achieved independent prescribing, in part, because groups like pharmacy and optometry had paved the way and persuaded the state authorities that non-medical prescribing was safe, effective and successfully contributed to the workforce redesign agenda. On the other hand, the case of the radiography profession reflects the opposite. As a profession that emerged and grew within the penumbra of medical authority, it endured a particularly difficult path towards independent prescribing, and the two branches of the profession achieved different outcomes as a result.

Radiography: allied to medicine or dependent upon it?

In the UK, radiography emerged in very different social circumstances to optometry. It emerged very much later, without the distinct and separate historical trajectory of optometry. Indeed, its history is intimately intertwined with that of the medical profession at the latter part of the 19th century, when X-rays were discovered and began to be used on a significant scale. As X-rays were only discovered in 1895 by a physicist in Germany, the profession of radiography has a far more recent history than that of optometry.

The use of contrast media to help explore the digestive system (and thus extend the application of X-rays beyond observations of bone structure) followed in 1904 as medical interest in the use of X-ray technology began to flourish (Larkin, 1983; Witz, 1992). Technological change at the dawn of the 20th century brought new specialities in medicine, such as anaesthetics and radiology, but these were at first regarded as marginal within medicine itself. It was a struggle for the speciality of radiology to establish itself within medicine, and thus its adherents were keen to reject claims of competence from any potential competitors in this fledging field of practice (Larkin, 1983; Witz, 1992).

Although many hospitals employed technicians to take X-rays and also comment on them, a clear division of labour separating the use of X-ray equipment to take pictures and the interpretation of these images (and the diagnosis) emerged early on. The creation of the Society of Radiographers in 1920 sought to agree it in a bid to establish its own niche in representing 'trained non-medical assistants' (Larkin 1983: 64). Thus, both radiologists and radiographers were intent upon establishing their own credentials as legitimate practitioners in their own spheres: radiologists as medical specialists and radiographers as qualified technicians, rather than purely lay technicians.

As the technology improved, so too did its use, and the First World War (1914–18) saw a large number of both doctors and orderlies rapidly trained and deployed (Larkin, 1983: 65). Shortly thereafter, the first formal qualification was made available to doctors wishing to specialise in radiology, and concern over orderlies returning from war service with radiographic skills prompted the BMA to firmly establish a distinction between those who operated the X-ray apparatus and those who interpreted the results and made the diagnosis.

At its inception, the new Society of Radiographers was dominated by medical doctors, some of whom who sat on its ruling council and who insisted that radiographers work under the direction and supervision of qualified medical practitioners. As it was also keen to secure medical support in its efforts to eliminate lay competition, it largely agreed, though internal disagreements over whether or not to concede over the right of radiographers to continue to report findings to radiologists caused consternation and further division within the Society (Larkin, 1983). Ultimately, however, the Society agreed to the revised scope of practice insisted upon by the medical profession, and contented itself with trying to raise the standards of its members within a restricted field of practice.

By 1936, the Society became an enthusiastic member of the Board of Registration of Medical Auxiliaries, firmly establishing its subordinate status and dependence upon medicine. It was only after a bid by the Society for Royal Charter status was opposed by the medical profession that the Society rejected the BMA's assertions that radiographic education should be controlled by medicine. Having openly opposed the views of the BMA, the Society's bid for a Royal Charter was rejected, sealing its domination by medicine. It was only in the later 1950s that it succeeded in escaping the yoke of medical dominance when it was able to work in tandem with other allied health professions to reject the restrictive terms of the Cope Report and lobby for recognition as a profession.

The state was persuaded to act by the collective rejection of the terms of the Cope Report by all the auxiliary professions (as the report sought to legally control medical auxiliaries), something they could not have hoped to achieve acting alone. In agreeing to a 'common front' in negotiations with the state, the allied health auxiliary professions achieved a leverage that would have been impossible without a unified approach (Larkin, 1983; Witz, 1992). Little changed in radiography until the 1970s, when more significant advances in technology demanded ever-increasing skills, and greater training and education requirements were developed (Hogg et al, 2007). After 1980, major developments in fields such as high-resolution computed tomography (CT), magnetic resonance imaging (MRI), positron emission tomography (PET) and ultrasound led to the establishment of advanced clinical roles within a postgraduate education framework, expanding the remit and role of the radiographer (Hogg et al, 2007). This included a radiographer reporting role in the wake of the NHS and Community Care Act 1990 (Hogg et al, 2007).

An advanced practitioner role was established, being recognised in the national career framework (Hogg et al, 2007). Consultant radiographer roles were finally established in 2003, following publication of the Department of Health's (2001) guidance on developing new allied health consultant positions (Kelly, 2008). It also led directly to the move towards radiography prescribing, which followed in 2005. Intriguingly, Yielder and Davis (2007) consider radiographers to be conformist, and tend even now to work in environments where tasks are protocol-driven and thus require less independent decision-making. For them, the workplace still comprises a culture in which radiographers are 'followers' rather than 'thinkers', suggesting an ongoing dependence on medicine.

Hardy et al (2008) explored the development of the advanced practitioner role in radiography across the UK, Australia and New Zealand, which all adopted similar educational qualifications at roughly the same pace, though the UK is thought to be slightly ahead in terms of role boundaries (Hardy et al, 2008). In Australia, radiography emerged in roughly parallel fashion, against a backdrop of medical control within a hierarchical division of labour. It followed a similar historical period of emergence following the discovery of X-rays and the subsequent medical application of the new technology in the early years of the 20th century. As in the UK, the early 'pioneer' radiographers were drawn from differing backgrounds (in Australia, they were apparently commonly referred to as 'skiagraphers') (Lewis, 2003). Lewis (2003) identified two types: those from the skilled labour market (physicists and electricians); and those from the unskilled labour market. Perhaps the best known was a Walter Filmer, a former railway engineer trained via an apprenticeship, who was subsequently appointed by a hospital board to be an 'honorary electrician and X-ray operator' as early as 1896. He and his brother were regarded as the first radiographers appointed at Newcastle Hospital in New South Wales (Smith, 2009).

To some extent, this reflects the same sort of division in early X-ray work found in the UK, where the 'technical' exponents of radiographic work (the electricians and physicists) felt themselves superior to the more caring-oriented X-ray nurses (Witz, 1992). Formal education did not begin until 1929 at a technical college in Melbourne. Although a number of state-based professional bodies already existed, it was not until 1947 that the Australian Institute of Radiography was established (which ultimately became the Australian Society of Medical Imaging and Radiation Therapy in 2016). Very quickly, it ceded authority over radiography education and autonomy to practise (agreeing to supervision by radiologists) to a conjoint board including the Royal Australian College of Radiologists, echoing similar criticisms of the UK profession (Witz, 1992).

Unlike the UK, radiography in Australia had largely been denied formal recognition as a full profession given that, as late as 1996, the Higher Education Council paper 'Professional education and credentialism' had implied that radiography belonged to the group it identified as 'semi-professions' (intriguingly, the document adopted definitions from the trait typology literature of Etzioni, Goode and Greenwood) (Lewis, 2003). This is even more striking given that optometry had attained degree status in 1992, comparable with the profession in the UK. However, this largely coincided with the dissolution of the conjoint board in 1987, thus ending the direct control over education exerted by radiology. Equally, the Australian profession did not attain the legislative recognition at the national level that its UK counterpart enjoyed, relying instead on rather piecemeal variants in state legislation, with no Act available at all in Western Australia at the time of Lewis's (2003) work.

The advent of the Australian NRAS in 2010 at last began to rectify this problem. For Lewis (2003), the link between the ongoing requirement for supervision by radiologists and access to Medicare rebates rendered radiography both subordinate to medicine and limited in scope by it. Thus, by its very nature, radiography (in both Australia and the UK) was subject to medical dominance almost at the outset, and its work was intimately linked to, and dependent upon, medicine throughout its existence.

As recently as 2007, calls for a greater role for Australian radiographers in areas such as 'descriptive' (technical) as opposed to 'medical' (diagnostic) reporting of radiographs was being tentatively recommended, considering the shortage of radiologists and the ageing population. Formalised recognition of the informal use of a 'red dot' system by radiographers, where they are able to flag suspected abnormalities to doctors, was one suggested solution (Smith and Baird, 2007). However, this arguably continues to acknowledge the limited role that radiographers play, and the way in which it is constrained and defined by radiologists.

These accounts help to make clear the distinct differences between the professions of optometry and radiography in their bids for recognition and professional status. While optometry forged its own path and achieved a modicum of success, arguing its case on its distinct scientific skills and knowledge, as well as its independent commercial practice, radiography was tied to medicine from the start and was willing to subordinate itself in order to legitimise its own niche within the sphere of medical control. Thus tied, it was only able to escape the clutches of medicine (partially, at least) by affiliating itself and its aims with the broader allied health bid for recognition and professional status. Optometry did not need to join the allied health collective, having achieved its own independent legislation. Thus, it is interesting to note how the contemporary profession negotiated its own move towards independent medicines prescribing rights – did it mirror that of optometry, or did it experience greater difficulty?

Radiography and the independent prescribing of medicines: divided and conquered?

The UK Crown Report (Department of Health, 1999) identified new forms of prescriber that would be drawn from the non-nursing and non-medical professions, and that would serve as part of the solution to the workforce shortfall in the NHS. It established two new forms of prescribing, reflecting the degree of independence each profession would be expected to adopt. Early candidates for independent prescribing included optometrists, physiotherapists and podiatrists; radiographers received no direct mention in the report, though the list of professions cited was not 'exclusive' (Department of Health, 1999: 50).

Shortly before the Crown Report, radiographers had already established the right to administer certain medicines via patient group directions (PGDs) (known as group protocols until 2000), which were largely used to manage treatment side effects in therapeutic care (oncology care) (Francis and Hogg, 2006). Indeed, in response to the Crown Report, the Society and College of Radiographers (SCoR) established a working party which agreed that prescribing would be necessary, particularly in the speciality areas of renography, radio-pharmaceuticals, contrast radiography and radiotherapy (Hogg and Hogg, 2003). At the time supplementary prescribing was approved for radiographers (the same time as for physiotherapists and podiatrists) in 2005, it was hailed as a useful means of working with patients with ongoing disorder where a diagnosis had already been made (Francis and Hogg, 2006).

In turn, this specific endorsement for therapeutic use implied that supplementary prescribing might be less than effective for diagnostic radiographers, and so it proved. Supplementary prescribing gave therapeutic radiographers substantial independence from physicians and circumvented the need to update obsolete PGDs, which also limited access to specific medicines at specific dosages, leaving little room for manoeuvre (Borthwick, 2008). However, a key requirement of supplementary prescribing has been the need to devise a clinical management plan (CMP) in conjunction with the physician, meaning that a diagnosis must be established first. Clearly, this has not been possible for diagnostic radiographers as their central role has always been designed to assist in establishing a diagnosis. On some occasions, for example, diagnostic radiographers might undertake serial imaging in bone densitometry and nuclear medicine, possibly over several years (in oncology work), but the frequency of the imaging may take place less than once a year, which would necessarily outdate the CMP, which must be reviewed annually (Hogg et al, 2007; Borthwick, 2008). Equally, most diagnostic imaging occurs in single examinations and is completed within six hours, rendering the use of supplementary prescribing largely irrelevant (Hogg et al, 2007; Borthwick, 2008). This suggested that diagnostic radiography might have a stronger case for independent prescribing than its therapeutic counterpart.

Yet, in 2016, the submission to the CHM to enable independent prescribing was accepted for therapeutic radiographers but rejected for diagnostic radiographers, essentially splitting the profession into two separate prescribing groups. Diagnostic radiographers play a central role in establishing diagnoses, which often involves administering medicines such as contrast agents (Borthwick et al, 2017). In these circumstances, PGDs are of limited value, and the resulting dependence on doctors to prescribe is complicated by a growing shortage of qualified radiologists (Borthwick et al, 2017).

One further feature is often overlooked in this scenario: should diagnostic radiographers become independent prescribers, they would be able to authorise patient-specific directions to other, non-prescribing, radiographers in order to enable them to administer the contrast agents or other medicines (Borthwick et al, 2017). This would further contribute to solving the workforce shortages and ensure a more flexible, interprofessional workplace environment. As most radiographers continue to work primarily in secondary care in hospitals, this would appear sensible, yet it was initially rejected. While therapeutic radiographers have finally been granted independent prescribing rights (in 2016), with a brief list of controlled drugs approved in 2019, diagnostic radiographers continue to be denied independent prescribing status (Borthwick et al, 2017).

Much of the opposition to radiography prescribing came from the Royal College of Radiologists during the public consultation exercise that preceded and informed the submission to the CHM. It relied upon a logic which stressed that overworked diagnostic radiographers would pose a threat to patient safety by having to take on these extra skills, and that the increasingly complex skills needed to take images via CT, MRI and radionuclide methods – the hybrid PET-CT/MRI – would demand greater technical competence (Royal College of Radiologists, 2015). In short, diagnostic radiographers were not to be burdened with extended scope of practice in prescribing, and exhorted to confine themselves to perfecting the techniques of clear and accurate image capture that would serve radiologists, who would then interpret the results and make a diagnosis (Royal College of Radiologists, 2015).

Discussion

Optometry and radiology constitute two clear examples of professions that may be regarded as established within contemporary mainstream healthcare. One has a long pre-modern history, with a degree of autonomy built on its claim to a unique knowledge base that is independent of medicine and a track record of retail business success; the other emerged firmly rooted in hospital practice comprising technicians competing with medicine within a medical sphere of practice. Optometry, historically male-dominated, was established prior to the advent of full medical hegemony and power; radiography, mainly female, arose within it. Yet, both continue to operate within limits to a scope of practice defined by the presence of two major medical specialities with which they closely interface: ophthalmology and radiology. Both groups have a clearly limited and subordinate role in the provision of healthcare within their own spheres, and both had to concede the right to make diagnoses within their fields of expertise. It is the latter that has so clearly influenced the limitations set on the prescribing of medicines for both groups, even in the current policy climate of workforce redesign and role flexibility.

Although the independent prescribing of medicines represents one of the core jurisdictions of medicine (Freidson, 1988), its exclusive control has been breached in the interests of sustainability in healthcare provision, with the interests of the state taking precedence over the wishes of the medical profession – but only to a degree. Medicine has still managed to limit the degree of independence in prescribing; indeed, 'independent prescribing' is only independent to a certain extent and does not equate to medical prescribing rights.

Unlike medical doctors, non-medical prescribers cannot prescribe most unlicensed medicines or controlled drugs, for example. Restrictions in the funding of non-medical prescribing roles in the NHS in the UK limit effectiveness, and access to the PBS in Australia is narrow and often excludes allied health prescribers (Borthwick et al, 2010). Thus, several subtle ways of exerting and limiting the developing scopes of practice of non-medical prescribers persist, even when legislation has been passed legitimising it.

The extent to which the broader managerialist agenda has had an impact on the professionalisation of optometry and radiography is more difficult to judge. Perhaps the reported tendency of radiographers to continue to conform to existing arrangements and accept medicine's cultural authority may have reduced its impact (Yielder and Davis, 2007). For example, following the introduction of consultant radiographer roles in 2003 in the UK, it has been suggested that their form of leadership emphasises primarily clinical skills within a narrow extension in scope of practice. While this involves, for example, making a report on a mammogram or ultrasound scan, it falls short of making a full diagnosis (Kelly et al, 2008). Equally, as a rule, consultant radiographers do not become managers, thus potentially reducing the influence on local or national service policy that managers might exert (Kelly et al, 2008).

The development of the Minor Eye Conditions Scheme (MECS) to support existing hospital eye services (managed by ophthalmologists) also illustrates the advances in optometry – but where specialist optometrists can only work with a high degree of autonomy within a limited scope of practice (Konstantakopoulou, 2018). In short, there is ample evidence to suggest that although allied health professions such as optometry and radiography have advanced in scope, responsibility and legitimacy in recent years, they nevertheless remain constrained by the power of the medical profession. Although it may be diminished as the medico-bureaucratic relationship has declined in the face of growing workforce pressures, it continues to exist in a modified but very real form.

What is evident and largely indisputable is the way in which these case exemplars demonstrate the utility of the theories drawn from the sociology of the professions. At the forefront is the neo-Weberian framework, which allows the strategies of the professions to be exposed to scrutiny, and the intensity of the jurisdictional and role boundary disputes to be clearly observed. Each profession expresses the nature of its professional project through its actions, its discourse and its relationships. Each seeks out powerful elites as allies (in the form of the state), and the outcome is reflective of the relative success of the sum of its strategies (Saks, 2015, 2016). Social closure was clearly practised most successfully by medicine; however, optometry and radiography engaged strategies of exclusion and usurpation as well. Attempts to secure a role in the treatment of eye disease by optometrists serves as an example of the latter, as was the bid for the independent prescribing of medicines by both professions. Bourdieuan theory also resonates through the contestation of professional titles in the desire to secure symbolic capital, for example, as manifest in the move from 'optician' to 'optometrist'. The dynamics of power, in a constant, ongoing, unending professional project, set in a competitive landscape, probably best captures the story of these allied health professions.

FOUR

Emerging allied health professions

The health professions are in a constant state of growth and evolution, with new professions continuing to emerge, many in response to new techniques and technologies, and being included under the umbrella of allied health. This chapter explores the emergent allied health occupations, that is, those groups that have recently achieved a level of consistency of title and organisation to then pursue professionalism.

Examples of occupations that have professionalised since the middle of the 20th century include exercise physiologists, rehabilitation counsellors, ODPs, DEs, genetic counsellors, perfusionists and sonographers. In 2020, AHPA introduced affiliate membership for a range of professions, including some emerging ones, for example, lymphoedema therapists, counsellors, diabetes educators, hand therapists, dermal clinicians, hearing aid audiologists, myotherapists, pedorthists, psychotherapists and spiritual counsellors. Not all these professions are recognised allied health professions in all jurisdictions.

A notable exception to the recognition of new allied health professions is the NHS. When the Professions Supplementary to Medicine Act 1960 was introduced, 12 professions were recognised. At the start of 2020, the NHS formally recognised 14 allied health professions: arts therapy, chiropody (now podiatry), dietetics, dramatherapy, medical laboratory sciences, music therapy, occupational therapy, orthoptics, physiotherapy, radiography, prosthetics and orthotics, speech and language therapy, clinical sciences, and paramedics (Larkin, 2002). Since 2005, just after the formation of the HPC, the recognised allied health professions in the UK have remained relatively stable. An important contribution of this chapter is the way that regulatory frameworks and funding structures influence the development of new professions.

There is limited published literature on the history and sociology of emerging professions. Some of the new professions (sonographers, perfusionists and genetic counsellors) have emerged as a direct response to new technologies. For example, perfusionists are responsible for operating the cardiopulmonary bypass machine during cardiac surgery, a technology that was first applied in the 1950s (Arsenault, 2000). Diagnostic sonography developed rapidly during the 1950s, and established the basis for the growth of the imaging profession (Hassall, 2007).

The dominant, largely neo-Weberian theories of professionalisation from the 20th century focused on the ways that occupational groups enhanced their status by staking a claim to a body of knowledge and preventing encroachment by others (Saks, 1983; Witz, 1992; Harrits, 2014). They achieved their exclusionary social closure by garnering state support to restrict access to education, credentials and opportunities to practise (Saks, 2010). By successfully lobbying the state, professional groups have been able to maintain various forms of legal monopoly, which gives them greater access to income, status and power (Macdonald, 1995; Currie et al, 2009). It is therefore understandable that emergent occupational groups are keen to secure their professional identity (Currie et al, 2009).

The features that distinguish an occupation from a profession are highly debated (Allsop and Saks, 2003). At the start of the 20th century, the medical profession was explicitly involved in the negotiation and shaping of the professional repertoires of many occupations (Larkin, 1983; Willis, 1983). Subsequently, the role of competing professions in shaping occupational jurisdictions has largely been replaced by the state and organisations through legislation and clinical governance.

During the middle of the 20th century, various scholars began to examine the way that occupational groups achieved professional status through organisation (Millerson, 1964; Wilensky, 1964; Etzioni, 1969). The term 'semi-profession' was coined to describe those occupational groups that did not fulfil the classical definition of a profession (doctors, lawyers and engineers), and contentiously (Witz, 1992) included teachers, nurses and social workers (Etzioni, 1969).

Wilensky (1964) proposed that professionalisation involved four stages, namely: doing something; achieving formal education; forming a professional association; and obtaining state support/endorsement/protection. This largely taxonomic approach has currency in the way that occupations approach the task of becoming a profession. At the same time, Millerson (1964) presented the concept of 'qualifying associations', which could be seen as the precursor structures for the development of formal professions. In addition to the aforementioned stages, Millerson included the maintenance of integrity through a code of conduct and that service be for the public good. Millerson later questioned these attributes, however, going on to say that to be recognised as a profession, the group must be 'subjectively and objectively' identified as a profession. In a similar vein to that proposed by Wilensky for the process of becoming a profession, the qualifying organisation established (in the absence of regulatory structures) parameters for entry to a profession, such as personal attributes, education and training, and experience, which could be seen as a form of social closure.

As several new allied health professions continue to emerge, the concept of a profession is probably more fluid at the commencement of the 21st century than it was over the past century, with several occupations claiming professional status. However, Larson's (1977) notion of the professional project still has currency. Larson proposed that specialist skills and expertise alone are not sufficient to attain higher status or market control. Achieving the professional project requires the collective input of the profession, even though not all members of the profession will be in support of the project, or indeed even aware of it (Larson, 1977; Macdonald, 1995). The following case studies illustrate that pursuit of the professional project involves access to university-degree credentials, state recognition through licensing or registration, the support of a professional association or the chartered status of professional bodies, and a unique and exclusive knowledge base and skills within the healthcare market.

However, these attributes are necessary but not sufficient for true professional recognition. Access to clients comes from endorsement by other professions who facilitate a patient pathway by making referrals and recommendations; and recognition by the state and other funders (such as insurers) increases access to funding. This suggests more than simply the achievement of certain requirements to enter a club, and some credibility by association.

Despite the variations in regulation across jurisdictions, the modern requirements for an occupation to enter and maintain the domain of a 'profession' appear to be rather consistent. In Australia, recognition by AHPA includes the following requirements of member professional groups (Allied Health Professions Australia, 2020, see: https://ahpa.com.au/):

- Tertiary health qualification at a level of at least Australian Qualifications Framework 7 (AQF7) (bachelor's degree level) or equivalent.
- Members are recognised to practise in mainstream government-funded health, disability, education, social and/or other systems or schemes.
- Practise within an evidence-based paradigm.
- Representation by a peak body with members in at least five Australian states or territories, and a constitution that specifies a national mandate.

Variations arise in the type of governing body involved in recognising, monitoring and enforcing these attributes. For instance, in Australia, there are several self-regulating professions that experience little interference from the state, with some receiving no state funding, while the UK NHS only recognises state-regulated allied health professions.

This chapter explores the way that allied health professions negotiate the professional landscape by examining the case studies of three occupational groups that are at different stages of their professionalisation journey: pedorthists, ODPs and DEs. We explore: the paths to professionalisation of each occupation; the processes of making the transition from a 'pre-profession' to a recognised profession; and the implications of making this transition in the late 20th and early 21st centuries.

The professionalisation of pedorthics

This case study focuses on the emerging professionalisation of pedorthics in the Australian context. The lack of written history about the profession means that much of the data for this case study was drawn directly from personal communication with key members of the profession in Australia, and their contacts internationally. We are particularly indebted to one of the key stakeholders involved in the professionalisation of the pedorthics profession in Australia, Karl-Heinz Schott, for his international, historic narrative of the profession.

Pedorthists are practitioners who modify and manufacture corrective and accommodative footwear, orthoses or other supportive devices to address conditions that affect the foot and mobility. Pedorthists can undertake foot assessments, including gait analysis and pressure testing, as well as make and modify a range of shoes, orthotics and foot-related devices. Several other professions are involved in the foot care division of labour, including podiatrists, chiropodists, foot care nurses and orthotists.

'Pedorthics' is a relatively new term, first coined in the US in the 1970s. While pedorthics is a relatively unknown profession, the function of pedorthists has been performed for centuries. The history of footwear manufacturers in Europe can be traced back at least a millennium to shoemaker guilds, and earlier to the cordwainer in around the 11th century (The Honourable Cordwainers' Company, 2020). Cordwainers were tradesmen with the skills to manufacture an entire shoe and were distinguished from cobblers who were shoe repairers (Mulligan, 1981). Shoemaking was an important occupation in many societies for millennia due to the general need for footwear among the population and the lack of industrial manufacturing processes until the 19th century. There is evidence that the shoemaking workforce was highly organised and had its own internal division of labour (Mulligan, 1981; The Honourable Cordwainers' Company, 2020).

The industrialisation and mechanisation of shoe manufacturing at the end of the 19th century meant that the craft of shoemaking was reduced to small numbers of specialised, niche craftsmen who targeted specific footwear needs, particularly shoe repairs and bespoke shoe manufacturing. Within this small group, some specialised further to make footwear for people with foot abnormalities and foot health problems.

The universal need for specialised and orthopaedic footwear means that the orthopaedic footwear manufacturer is a recognised occupation in many countries. For instance, the Japanese have an orthopaedic technician course. In Central Europe, as the field of medical orthopaedics developed, some shoemakers worked alongside orthopaedic surgeons to provide medical footwear, subsequently establishing subgroups of orthopaedic shoemakers and shoemaker guilds. The focus on orthopaedic footwear increased after the First World War in response to the number of injured servicemen with foot and mobility problems. As with other allied health professions, the limited available history is largely written from an Anglo–American perspective, so there is little published literature on the international evolution of this workforce.

In the UK, footwear services are managed by prosthetics and orthotics allied health professionals and there has been no separation into pedorthics. In the US, the guild system was not established in the same way or with the same strength as it was in Europe. When industrial-scale footwear manufacturing was introduced, former shoemakers became shoe repairers. The pedorthic profession in the US evolved from the need for shoe repairers and retailers to modify footwear for medical purposes, with the formation of the first professional association in 1958, which subsequently became the American Board for Certification of Orthotics, Prosthetics and Pedorthics in 2007.

The pedorthics profession is relatively small internationally, with around 600 certified pedorthists in Canada and around 750 in the US. Pedorthics training in the US is fully vocational to the level of certificate or diploma.

The term 'pedorthist' and the associated profession have evolved in Australia over the past three decades. Early discussion around the use of the term 'pedorthics' in Australia dates back to the early 1990s at the conference of the Australian Surgical and Orthopaedic

Footwear Makers Association. Some practitioners are believed to have then adopted the term 'pedorthist' to describe their role, despite the absence of formal recognition of that title. In 1998, the association renamed itself the 'Australian Medical Grade Footwear Association Incorporated'. The term 'pedorthist' was first formally introduced in 2007 in Australia, when the professional association was named the 'Australian Pedorthic Medical Grade Footwear Association'. In 2013, the current title of the 'Pedorthic Association of Australia' was registered.

The evidence of the organisation of the early Australian pedorthists is anecdotal but the bootmakers and later the shoe repairer's associations are believed to have held annual conferences from the early 1960s. The formation of an independent association for orthopaedic footwear manufacturers was initiated at the 1972 Shoemakers Conference in Brisbane.

Initially, a large proportion of custom surgical bootmakers were employed in public hospitals, the Repatriation, Artificial Limb and Appliance Centres (RALAC) until their closure in 1995, and in the then named 'Societies for Crippled Children' (now known as 'Northcott'). The public sector was a large employer of pedorthists, at that stage due to the needs of war veterans and people with polio. More recently (since the mid-1990s), the employment of pedorthists has shifted to employment in private clinics, with relatively few employed in larger, public organisations. This may be a response to changing population needs, with fewer war veterans and young people with disabilities from conditions such as polio. Instead, pedorthists are more likely to provide services for people with disabilities and chronic illness (such as diabetes), with their services funded by insurers and individual patients. There are no data available to determine the exact distribution of the profession in Australia, but the high proportion of practitioners in private practice is believed to reflect the international employment structure of pedorthists.

Since their formal organisation as an occupational group, pedorthists have continually evolved their training pathways. Initially, surgical bootmakers trained in an apprenticeship alongside the limb maker (later known at the prosthetist) and splint maker (later known as the orthotist). The last vocational surgical footwear course at Sydney College of Technical and Further Education School of Footwear ended in the early 2000s. The Pedorthics Association of Australia commenced its certification training programme in 2002 (Certificate in Pedorthics and a Certificate in Manufacturing [CPedCM]). Entry to the programme required the applicant to have 200 days of relevant work experience and to have completed another trade or a tertiary educational qualification. The structured programme was delivered and managed by the Australian School of Pedorthics and included: an online theoretical component, including some content and examinations from the US; face-to-face theoretical lectures and workshops; lectures and workshops on pedorthic manufacturing; a retail shoe-fitting programme, which was assessed through competencies; and the custom production of specialised boots, which were assessed against a theoretical and technical competency framework. After five years of direct pedorthic work experience, the applicant is eligible for assessment by the certification panel. On successful completion, the candidate is admitted to the Pedorthic Register (Australian Pedorthists Registration Board [see: www.aprb.org.au/]). There are three levels of certification of pedorthists in Australia: CPedCM, pedorthic retailers and certified pedorthists. Certified pedorthists undertake shoe modifications and make custom accommodative foot orthoses but do not manufacture shoes.

The pedorthic profession was keen to move into university-based training to increase the quality of the education programme and to achieve equivalence with other healthcare professionals. A shift into higher education also provided the occupation with an opportunity to undertake much-needed research to create a scientific basis for their work.

The relatively small numbers in the profession, and specialised equipment requirements, meant that the introduction of a training programme was expensive. To cover the capital costs, the Pedorthic Association of Australia partnered with a large international supplier of orthopaedic footwear machinery to create a joint commercial/ training hub for the profession and to act as the Australian base for the manufacturer. In 2015, the first students of the three-year Bachelor of Pedorthics graduated from Southern Cross University, setting the new educational entry standard for registration as a CPedCM.

Pedorthists are registered by the Australian Pedorthic Registration Board. They are responsible for: certifying pedorthists; accrediting and reviewing training facilities for pedorthists; monitoring and upholding codes of conduct or ethics approved by the Pedorthic Association of Australia; and allocating continuing professional development points to pedorthists. Only pedorthists who are registered with the Australian Pedorthists Registration Board are eligible to access certain forms of funding; therefore, this is a form of co-regulation (Australian Health Ministers' Advisory Council, 2018). Co-regulation involves a self-regulating body entering into an agreement with a third party, such as the state or another funder, that recognises the endorsement of the self-accrediting body and provides additional benefits (such as payment) to the self-accrediting practitioners.

Pedorthists do not have state protection of their title; however, the high cost of entry to the profession due to the high capital outlay and the high cost of the products they produce (sometimes several thousands of dollars) would be a strong disincentive to competitors. Limiting state funding to those practitioners who are registered with the Australian Pedorthists Registration Board effectively excludes others from access to funding and service provision.

This model of professional self-regulation is a kind of 'private ordering', which bestows benefits on the practitioners and their clients that would not normally be available through the laws of contract and employment (Lester, 2016). While this relationship is largely removed from state involvement and endorsement, it still conforms to the neo-Weberian concept of social closure because membership to the 'club' provides benefits, status and access to resources that are unavailable to non-members (Parkin, 1979; Saks, 2012, 2016).

The pedorthists have implemented self-regulation as a way to 'put in place, operate and gain acceptance for standards and processes that are designed to ensure quality of practice' (Lester, 2016). Self-regulation ensures that certified members are positioned as the sole providers of pedorthic services to several government and private insurers. This restriction of market access is a further form of monopoly over their services and reinforces both the value and the status of professional closure. While other practitioners may provide similar services, their lack of formal endorsement limits their market access and their external credibility.

In 2020, Australia had 45 certified members on the Pedorthic Register, of whom 28 were CPedCM. Each pedorthist employs a non-certified workforce of approximately two or three support staff, who may be technical, retail or administration support staff. The size of this workforce is unknown.

The pedorthic profession represents a remnant, and specialist niche, of what was formerly a large, well-organised artisan occupation. The small numbers who have retained the skills of footwear production following the industrialisation of footwear manufacturing have divided into medical and non-medical branches. Those in the medical branch of footwear manufacturing are particularly niche. They have had to self-organise into an occupational group and establish internal training standards, which were initially vocational but have more recently moved into the university sector (in Australia at least).

As an ancient craft-based occupation, it is valuable to make some comparisons with other similar disciplines, such as optometry. Like pedorthics, the art of making spectacles and the understanding of optics also has ancient origins (Enoch, 2006). Both occupations have long histories of organisation into guilds (Larkin, 1983).

Like optometry, pedorthics is a technical profession with a long history that was affected by changes in technology at the end of the 19th century (lens making and machines to make shoes). However, this is where the similarities end. A key difference in the occupations is that spectacles are almost wholly produced to correct a defect in eyesight. In other words, spectacles are predominantly a health-related product. In contrast, footwear is predominantly a commercial fashion product and only a small proportion of those products require custom manufacture or modification to respond to health problems. Consequently, optometrists or opticians took some level of ownership over the medical aspects of their technology (spectacles), resulting in a strengthening and early professionalisation of their occupation. Pedorthists are a small group of practitioners who have embraced the health aspects of the commercial product (shoes) and only recently created a healthcare profession from it. Additionally, there is a strong and long scientific history behind lens manufacturing and the production of eyewear. Despite (or perhaps because of) the complexity of footwear, it remains much more of an art than a science (Ahmed et al, 2020).

Changing population health has been an important driver for the nature and distribution of pedorthists' work. The eradication of polio in Australia by the mid-20th century coincided with an increase in chronic illness. Instead of managing the long-term complications associated with diseases like polio, the pedorthic profession has had to adapt to a growing population of people with complications arising from conditions such as diabetes, which causes foot ulceration and foot deformity, and can lead to amputation. As the prevalence of diabetes and other chronic illnesses increases, it is likely that the demand for pedorthic services will also increase. Also, unusually, the risks and severity of the conditions treated by the profession are likely to increase, demanding an increased scientific basis for the activities of the profession.

Like the optometry profession, pedorthists now have access to rapid and significant improvements in technology. Examples include 3D scanning and printing technologies that facilitate the scanning of a foot or limb and the manufacture of a shoe remote from where the scan took place. The technology has the advantages of being able to simplify manufacturing, as well as separating the patient assessment from the point of production, creating potential for devices to be manufactured offshore with lower production costs. This separates the manufacturer from the assessor (the engineer from the technician). The longer-term impacts of technology on the profession remain to be seen. As highlighted earlier in this book, the ability of machine learning to replicate professional expertise has the potential to replace the 'indeterminacy' component of the pedorthist's role (Jamous and Peloille, 1970). However, footwear is a highly complex intervention because of the interplay of foot pathology, foot dynamics and foot morphology with variations in shoe technology and patient preferences; therefore, it is likely that this process will take some time.

The professionalisation of operating department practitioners

ODPs (as they are known in the UK), or operating theatre practitioners or technicians (Australia), assist surgeons and anaesthetists in the operating theatre. Their roles can include preparing and maintaining an operating theatre and its equipment, assisting the surgical team during operations, and supporting patients in the recovery room (Timmons and Tanner, 2004). An important sociological commentator on the ODP role and professionalisation is Stephen Timmons (Timmons and Tanner, 2004, 2008; Timmons, 2011), and his work is cited extensively in this case study.

ODPs are an example of an occupational group at different stages of transition internationally. In the UK, ODPs were one of the most recent professions to achieve professional closure through registration with the HPC (in 2004) and are a recognised allied health profession. In contrast, in Australia, this group of workers lack a nationally recognised consistent title, and at the time of writing, there were no formal training or career pathways for ODPs.

There are some other interesting aspects of the ODP workforce. Relatively unusually for allied health professions, ODPs are exclusively employed in hospitals (Timmons, 2011; Corbett and Suckling, 2018). Typically, other allied health professions are employed in a wide range of settings and can practise autonomously. A second interesting consideration is that despite ODPs being classified as allied health professions in the UK since 2017 (NHS England, 2017), their roles most closely align with, and are often in direct competition with, the nursing profession (Timmons and Tanner, 2004; Corbett and Suckling, 2018). As a result of these differences in stages of professionalisation in different jurisdictions, the ODP is an interesting occupation to study from the perspective of an emerging profession and the role of the state in supporting professionalisation.

The precursor to the ODP appears to be the theatre technician, which was developed in cooperation with the BMA in the 1940s (Timmons and Tanner, 2004). They first received formal recognition as an occupational group in the UK NHS in 1970 as an organisational and managerial response to addressing surgical waiting lists. According to Timmons, the role was first proposed as a technician role that would receive in-house training (Timmons and Tanner, 2004). It is notable that this role was developed under the stewardship of the BMA and not with the support of the nursing profession given that it appears to be closely aligned with the role of the theatre nurse. Their transition to a registered profession in 2004 was also a fortuitous response to workforce shortages. At the time of the formation of the HPC in 2002, eight other professions were also pursuing the process of professionalisation.

Prior to registration with the HPC, the professional Association of Operating Department Practitioners (AODP) had established a voluntary register. Like the self-regulation of pedorthists, the register imposed a degree of occupational closure, which meant that the NHS was required to employ only ODPs on the register. The exclusive employment of registered practitioners by the NHS amounted to social closure. However, the AODP, as with several other occupational groups, perceived that the ultimate sign of professional closure was recognition by the state in the form of state regulation. Consistent with the pursuit of the professional project, the AODP actively pursued the upgrading of their qualifications from a vocational award to a university-based diploma and the replacement of their professional newsletter with an academic journal. Their single professional register placed them in a strong position with the HPC in comparison with the other, less unified, professions seeking HPC regulation.

The AODP pursued regulation to improve patient care but other goals of regulation were largely to benefit the profession, including parity with other professions (particularly nurses), increased pay and better career opportunities. The ODPs also expected that regulation with the HPC would ensure access to controlled medications; however, the legislation to enact that change took some time to introduce after regulation.

According to Timmons's (2011) analysis, not all members of the profession agreed with the pursuit of HPC regulation. Concerns related to the increasing educational demands and the growing gap between the vocationally trained members of the profession and the more recent diploma graduates. A further concern was the cost of regulation to the members. This supports Larson's (1977) observation that while professional support is essential to achieve the professional project, not all members of the profession will be supportive.

Following the achievement of regulation, the function of the AODP was called into question. Previously, the association had been the regulator of the profession but this function was now overtaken by the HPC. Members already unwilling to pay for regulation with the HPC were reluctant to pay additional fees for membership of their professional association, whose role was in question. Ironically, the AODP, which had pushed so hard for professional regulation, ceased operation in 2006 due to financial insolvency as a result of their regulatory success.

The benefits of regulation to the ODPs were questionable. As their work is largely controlled by the NHS, there were no additional pay benefits to the ODPs, and it is unclear how they would negotiate a more competitive position. Shortly after regulation was achieved, the NHS common pay scale, 'Agenda for Change', was introduced, which provided competency-based pay and largely levelled the playing field for NHS employed staff (Department of Health, 2004a). This brought ODP pay on a par with nursing.

Timmons (2011) proposes that one of the most important drivers to achieve regulation was the professional competition between the ODPs and nurses. This point was addressed later by Corbett and Suckling (2018), who examined the 'credential creep' of ODPs in the UK NHS. Having achieved professional regulation through membership of the HPC, members of the ODP profession agitated to increase their qualification from a diploma to degree-level training. Corbett and Suckling present data suggesting that this is because the ODPs felt threatened by nursing roles, and percieved that if they were not equally qualified, then their roles could be at risk by the more 'predatory' nursing profession.

Timmons succinctly summarises the key issues arising from this case study. This case study challenges the assumption that the path to professionalisation brings increased benefits to every occupational group. Indeed, given the dominance of the state as both a monopoly employer and regulator of the ODPs, there was little room for any manoeuvring on behalf of the profession in terms of their role, status or pay. Importantly, as Timmons points out, the ODPs had effectively already achieved professional closure prior to the introduction of state regulation. The introduction of regulation was an additional bureaucratic burden but with no additional accompanying benefits for the profession.

The ODPs lacked a unique professional jurisdiction that was distinct from the medical division of labour or nursing. As a relatively low-risk profession, the benefits of regulation to the state are unclear in this case given that regulation is meant to protect the public and ensure quality standards. Timmons suggests that regulation may be a state-mediated way of extending control over professional groups; however, it is far more likely that local clinical governance would be a better measure of quality for this group given the hospital contexts in which they work.

The professional pathway of developmental educators in the disability field

DEs are a small, relatively new allied health profession that has developed in South Australia in response to the changing models of disability service provision. They are the first formally recognised and registered allied health profession group in Australia specifically dedicated to disability.

DEs create strategies to support the individual developmental learning goals of people with challenges such as acquired brain injury, physical and neurological disabilities, autism spectrum disorders, intellectual disability, and other disabilities. They also work closely with families and caregivers, as well as other allied health professionals who may be involved in the support of an individual. DEs are a self-regulated profession, registered by Developmental Educators Australia Incorporated (DEAI) (see: www.deai.com.au/).

As with the other emerging professions, there is limited published literature on the history or sociology of DEs, though the history has been chronicled by the DEAI and briefly by Ellison and Matthews (2012). Most of the information presented in this case study has been provided by the DEAI (Developmental Educators Australia Incorporated, 2020).

Unusually for an emerging profession, DEs have a relatively short pre-professional history because of the emergence of their role in response to the shift from a medical model to a social model in the management of people with disability in Australia from the 1980s. Attitudes to people with disability began to change in response to the needs of returned servicemen after the First and Second World Wars; however, the move towards deinstitutionalisation did not commence in Australia until the 1980s (Butteriss, 2012). This shift recognised the interaction between the person with a disability and the societal barriers that prevented them from participating fully. The change is reflected in the rejection of language like 'mental retardation' to 'intellectual and developmental disability'.

The states and not-for-profit organisations were initially responsible for the delivery of the majority of disability services, resulting in an array of inconsistent approaches and models (Productivity Commission, 2011). It was not until the introduction of the NDIS in 2013 by the then Labor government, which first commenced in 2016, that disability services had a stable and centralised commonwealth funding and service approach (Buckmaster and Clark, 2018). The changing disability landscape was accompanied by incremental and sporadic policy changes at the state and commonwealth levels, which have been reflected in different challenges to the professionalisation of the DE role.

Between 1976 and 2006, people with intellectual disabilities were supported in South Australia by the South Australian Intellectual Disability Services Council (IDSC). The IDSC was responsible for planning and providing support and advocacy services for people with intellectual disabilities and their families. In 2006, the IDSC became part of the government department Disability SA (George and George, 2014).

Prior to a restructure of the IDSC in the 1980s, most community-based services for people with intellectual disabilities were delivered by registered mental deficiency nurses. There is little documentation about mental deficiency nurses in Australia; however, the title has been used in the UK since 1919 (Mitchell, 2019). Mental deficiency nurses were largely associated with the provision of institutional care for people with intellectual disabilities (Mitchell, 2019).

The restructure of the IDSC reflected the move towards the deinstitutionalisation of people with intellectual disability and resulted in the development of regional teams, whose role included case management, community development and developmental programming. To support this change in care ethos and philosophy, a new approach to the management of people with disabilities was developed in South Australia through the collaboration of academics from Flinders University, executives from the IDSC and the non-government sector, and disability professionals. The philosophy underpinning the professional training of DEs in South Australia drew from two, sometimes opposing, ideologies of normalisation and applied behaviour analysis (Emerson and McGill, 1989).

The result of the collaboration was the introduction of a two-year Diploma of Developmental Disabilities in the late 1980s, taught at what was then Sturt College. When Sturt College amalgamated with Flinders University in 1991, a three-year Bachelor of Applied Science – Developmental Disabilities was created, which marked the beginning of the professional training of DEs.

Registered mental deficiency nurses did not meet the requirements for the reconfigured service. They were encouraged to supplement their training with formal studies in disability, specifically, the Diploma in Developmental Disabilities.

The course title changed several times over the next decade to respond to the needs presented by various restructures of the IDSC. In the mid-1990s, an organisational restructure within the IDSC saw DEs become 'options coordinators'. This change, as well as the changes to the degree title, saw the use of the title 'developmental educator' reduced significantly, with 'disability professional' being the preferred terminology. In early 2000, the degree was rebadged as the Bachelor of Disability and Community Rehabilitation.

The next two decades were a challenging time for the professionalisation of the disability workforce as they struggled to clarify their own identity within a changing policy and funding landscape. The Developmental Educators Association (DEA) was established in South Australia in the early 1990s and developed the first code of ethics and practice in 1994. It was the first professional body to support the development of the profession of developmental education. Due to a lack of membership, eligibility was broadened to capture a wider field of professionals working in disability. The association changed its name to 'Disability and Rehabilitation Professionals Association' (DaRPA). DEs continued to be represented on the committee with a strong interest in their profession. In 2008, a group called Australian Disability Professionals (ADP) formed to become a national representative body of professional activities within the disability sector. It later entered into a collaboration with New Zealand colleagues, becoming the 'Australasian' body in 2010 (Ellison and Matthews, 2012). DaRPA joined ADP in 2009. ADP ceased operation in 2012. It is unclear why the ADP ceased operation; however, it coincided with the introduction of the National Disability Scheme, which was in the process of bringing together national disability services and organisations (National Disability Scheme, 2013).

Two key and related activities occurred that helped consolidate the professional profile of the DE in South Australia. The first was the formation of DEAI in 2009. The DEAI was introduced to address the lack of recognition, poor employment outcomes, limited career options and a lack of sense of belonging to a profession for DEs. The formation of the DEAI received the support of the public sector union, the South Australian Public Services Association. The DEAI incorporated in 2010 after a year of planning. The DEAI established clear criteria for full membership to the association and established the standards for the educational qualifications required to be a practising DE.

The second key development for the professionalisation of DEs was their recognition as allied health professionals by the South Australian

Commissioner for Public Sector Employment (2011). Prior to this, DEs in government were employed in the 'operational stream', which did not require a professional qualification. DEs were able to seek reclassification from the operational to the allied health stream based on their qualification from 2011. In response, Flinders University changed the title of the degree to Bachelor of Disability and Developmental Education (BDDE) in order to better align with the professional title of its graduates.

The BDDE is a multidisciplinary degree with input from a range of professional disciplines, such as psychology, speech pathology, occupational therapy, social work, education and physiotherapy. Several other professionals work in the disability field, including occupational therapists, speech and language therapists, psychologists, physiotherapists, educators, and social workers. All of these professions have input into the DE training programme. The differentiating feature of DEs is the specialised and comprehensive knowledge they gain about disability during their four years of tertiary training: models, concepts, values and attitudes, ethics, and especially positive behaviour support training. In particular, they achieve core competencies around the professional practice of and identity as a DE, alongside a contemporary understanding of disability theory and human diversity.

Only professionals with 'disability studies' qualifications (bachelor/master) recognised by the DEAI can call themselves a DE. As with other self-regulating professions, there is no legislated protection of the title; however, in recognition of the co-regulation status, only members of the DEAI are eligible for certain government-funded disability services (such as some of the services funded by the NDIS). This effectively provides a form of professional closure for DEs.

The DEAI has identified that a challenge for the profession has been the lack of clearly defined professional boundaries. Many DEs refine their skills and expertise in the workplace through their practice and professional development, and the scope of practice is largely defined by the needs of the clients and the contexts in which DEs work. The DEAI is yet to create a set of scope of practice documents to provide better guidance to DEs (and other professions); however, they have established a set of core competencies and skills within those. The practice of DEs is guided by the 'Code of conduct' and the DEAI (2015) 'Code of ethics and practice for DEs' (see: www.deai.com.au/about/about-code-of-ethics).

Despite the plurality of the DE role, there has been little resistance to its development from other professions. When the NDIS was first rolled out, there was some competition between practitioners for 'billable hours'. The main challenge of the DEs has been to achieve recognition from other professions for their specific skill set. The profile of the profession is gradually increasing and is associated with an increase in the number of new positions for DEs. This is particularly the case for South Australia as this is where most DEs practise. Ellison and Matthews (2012) suggest that a lack of understanding of the role of the DE by the public and other professions has potentially reduced its standing as a profession. In particular, they suggest that some perceive the role to be associated with 'minding' people, rather than providing an expert technical skill set.

DEs are still predominantly based in South Australia, even though the DEAI recognises relevant professional qualifications in disability from universities in other states. The relatively small size of the profession means that it remains little known outside South Australia. The DEAI continues to explore various pathways to achieving this. For example, as well as individual course accreditation, the DEAI offers professional accreditation for university disability studies degrees: universities that offer a bachelor- or master-level disability studies degree and who are interested in professional accreditation by the DEAI can complete the University Disability Studies Degree Accreditation Application. The introduction of the NDIS has seen a growth in interest in the DE role, as well as a significant increase in membership.

Other states have also attempted to professionalise roles associated with the disability sector, including the 'social trainer' in Tasmania and Western Australian, and the 'programme officer' in Queensland (Ellison and Matthews, 2012). However, the lack of standardised training across the range of programmes limits the ability of these groups to develop a consistent professional identity.

The DEAI has sought membership with the national peak body for allied health professions, AHPA; however, AHPA now requires membership with the National Alliance for Self Regulated Health Professions (NASRHP) as a prerequisite for entry. The DEAI is currently pursuing membership of the NASRP. The DEAI recognises that they will have to consider the costs involved and balance this against the outcomes from such membership.

The development of the DE role reinforces the pathway to professionalisation, that is, identifying a need, establishing a strong professional association, creating a degree-level course and obtaining government support and, in this case, funding. This case study illustrates several interesting points. The first is the identification of the DEs as allied health professionals. The contemporary disability movement is defined as a social model, rather than a medical model, and, indeed, largely rejects the medical model. The growth of the disability movement, particularly over the past decade in Australia, has seen increased focus and funding in this field. Indeed, the introduction of a NDIS replaces pockets of block-grant-based funding, which limited the opportunities for professional (and probably technical) innovation and hierarchies. While there have been several attempts at creating a professional tier of the disability workforce, professionalisation of the DEs was enabled by strong state-level support, and has been enhanced by the increased demand created by the introduction of the nationally funded NDIS.

However, given that the disability movement is relatively new, there has not been access to a recognised professionalisation pathway for the disability workforce outside a management framework. The DE sits across health, social care and education. Education has an established professional framework but tends to only work in the educational setting, whereas allied health practitioners can practise autonomously and move across a range of different settings and contexts, and continue to be recognised and rewarded for their professional title. In other words, allied health provided a ready-made pathway to professionalisation for the DEs that was not available in the disability context.

Leicht and Fennell (2001) highlight the challenges to professionalisation faced by occupations that deal with stigmatised groups of patients, such as the elderly, people with infectious disease and the mentally ill. Occupations dealing with more stigmatised patients face more challenges to professionalisation than those that deal with so-called 'heroic' interventions or highly technical procedures. Therefore, given that the DE role was specifically designed to meet the needs of people with disability, and grew out the stigmatised field of 'mental retardation', their professionalisation as an allied health profession is noteworthy. It is also a highly feminised profession group.

The pathway to professionalisation largely followed neo-Weberian principles (Parkin, 1979; Saks, 1983, 2010, 2013). The market for the professionalisation of the disability workforce emerged from the changes and growth in the disability sector, supported by state-based policies and funding. The DEs first had to create a philosophical framework to guide their practice, and this was codified into a training course. The new philosophy of practice and the training requirement effectively defined the task domain and established a new boundary around the scope of practice, or social closure (Parkin, 1979), and was associated with a specified client group.

While the DE could have been seen to be usurping the role of the registered 'mental retardation' nurse, the cessation of that role was effectively driven by the state as a result of the new philosophies underpinning disability services. The DEAI imposed a level of social exclusion by establishing minimum entry criteria (credentials), while membership of the DEAI provides a form of social closure by limiting access to government funding to registered members. The DEs were able to achieve social closure through strong professional identity, state support and co-regulation, whereas attempts by members of the disability workforce to professionalise in other states failed because of a lack of clear professional identity.

The demise of the registered 'mental retardation' nurse is also noteworthy. Little is written about 'unsuccessful professions'. However, the ability for these workers to transition to DEs could be seen as an evolutionary step. Similar changes have been noted in the development in community psychiatric nursing, with changes associated with modifications to the treatment and management of mental health (Godin, 1996).

Discussion

This chapter illustrates several key points about the professionalisation of allied health. The first is that the allied health umbrella creates opportunities for new professions to emerge to respond to specific areas of societal needs. The examples of pedorthists and DEs demonstrate the evolution of relatively small, niche areas of practice that have responded to changes in population demographics and social change, such as attitudes to disability. The state, in collaboration with universities, has provided support through the funding of higher education programmes that produce graduates to meet those needs. For the DEs, allied health provided a pathway and a framework for professionalisation that was not available in the disability sector.

The second point is the value of self-regulation (or, specifically, co-regulation) to create legitimacy for those professions. The self-regulation pathway ensures that the members of the profession adhere to an agreed set of standards, where co-regulation – that is, the provision of state funding only to those practitioners who meet the self-regulation standards – effectively creates market closure for those members of the profession.

An apparent distraction for health profession groups is the desire to achieve state-endorsed professional closure; however, except for the protection of their professional title, there appears to be little else to gain from state regulation. The factors that detracted from the achievement of the respective professional projects appear to come from a lack of clear professional identity and focus, and a lack of coordinated leadership. In the example of the DEs, some the challenges to professional identity were created by the rapidly evolving policy landscape as these were largely the tools for defining and implementing disability practice.

While the pedorthic profession and the DEs did not achieve their professionalisation in a linear or necessarily efficient path, the lessons from their approaches to professionalisation could be adopted to support the more efficient introduction of other new professions. The pathway to successful professionalisation is largely reflected in Larson's (1977) concept of the professional project, and codified in the entry standards for the National Alliance of Self Regulating Health Professions and the Australian Health Practitioners Register. These include: clarity around the scope of practice; an organised professional body with agreed standards; a code of ethics/practice and/or professional conduct; competency standards and course accreditation; internal quality management systems, such as complaints procedures and continuing professional development; recency of practice; and practitioner certification requirements (National Alliance of Self Regulating Health Professions, 2020).

A further consideration is the role of the state in mediating new professions. This chapter has juxtaposed a largely free-market approach (pedorthists in Australia) with an almost wholly state-run model of healthcare organisation (the NHS), which is intricately bound with regulation, and a state-mediated approach in terms of the DEs. The latter developed predominantly from changing state requirements and is heavily reliant on state funding.

From the perspective of allied health evolution, a state monopoly on health services presents challenges for new professions to enter the market. This is illustrated by the proliferation of allied health professions in Australasia and North America that have not achieved recognition in the UK market. Some examples include exercise physiologists, diabetes educators, pedorthists and rehabilitation counsellors. It is unclear whether these functions are provided by others within the NHS. In contrast, the more pluralistic model of healthcare delivery in Australia means that professionalism is largely open to occupational groups that meet the requirements of a self-regulating profession and that can convince the public or funders to purchase their services. Once a profession has achieved professional status through self-regulation, they have a stronger chance of convincing the state to employ them in state-funded organisations. Exercise physiologists are a good example of a profession that achieved professional closure through self-regulation in the last 30 years and is now employed in public hospitals and community settings.

The traditional assumption proposes that only the state can license or create professions. However, as the case of the pedorthists has illustrated, while the state has certainly been a purchaser of pedorthic services (directly through hospitals and indirectly through insurers, such as Veterans Affairs), their route to professionalisation has largely been driven by the profession, independent from the state. The model of self-regulation adopted by the profession occurred without state intervention or endorsement. However, self-regulation by the profession was sufficient to convince the funders and purchasers of services that only registered pedorthists are eligible for reimbursement for their services, effectively providing them with a privileged position over non-registered practitioners. In other words, self-regulation has provided a social bargain with the public that bestows privileges on the profession in return for upholding transparent quality standards. This model has enabled the development of a new profession in an open-market economy. It is interesting to note the lack of differentiation of the pedorthic workforce from the prosthetic and orthotic workforce in the UK NHS.

A further consideration is the value of professionalisation to both the profession and the public. Professionalisation of the pedorthic profession, as achieved through professional closure, has clearly provided benefits to the profession and the public. The roles of the pedorthic profession itself are relatively low-risk, and certainly do not warrant protection by the state; however, endorsed quality standards will provide some level of certainty and protection to the public.

The value of professionalisation of the ODP is less clear. It is a relatively low-risk profession that works in a highly structured and regulated organisational environment. The quest for professionalisation has placed upward pressure on credentials, and therefore increased the cost of training an ODP. What was initially introduced as an auxiliary profession has evolved into a direct competitor to nursing (Larkin, 2002; Timmons and Tanner, 2004). There is no explicit monopoly over a body of knowledge that shapes the practice of the ODP, and the quality of their care is likely to be managed through local supervisory relationships. Except for the protection of professional title, there are no material benefits to the regulation of this workforce.

The third point is the cost of professionalisation. In all case studies, the ODPs, DEs and pedorthists experienced 'credential creep' to maintain their professional position. For both the ODPs and the pedorthists, increasing their training was an explicit strategy to maintain their professional status and to provide parity with their peers (other allied health practitioners and nursing) (Corbett and Suckling, 2018). However, credential creep leads to an increase in the cost of training a professional, in this case, with no increase in salary. There are additional costs associated with the regulation of practitioners. What we see is an increasing cost to attain and sustain 'professional' status that is borne both directly by the professionals and indirectly by the purchasers of their services in the form of higher costs. There has been no economic analysis of the cost of professionalisation of the allied health professions; however, an analysis of the professionalisation of the nursing profession highlights the issues of higher training costs and subsequent wage pressures on what has become a higher-status profession as a result of professionalisation (Francis, 1999). The costs of professionalisation, including training and regulation, need to be seen in the context of the societal benefits and the risks of the work being undertaken.

Credential creep is a feature of several allied health professions, which have shifted from three-year to four-year undergraduate and postgraduate training methods. The credential creep also benefits higher education providers who are also seeking to maintain their market share in an increasingly competitive environment.

Olofsson (2016) argues that the number of new students studying vocational programmes has altered the relationship between the higher education system and occupation-professional categories. While the expansion of the university sector has created opportunities for students to be directed into different types of jobs, formal training for professions has also increased 'due to changes in the economy and to decisions by the state to increase the formal training for an increasing number of occupations and semi-professions' (Olofsson, 2016, p.2). Universities are linking their programmes to existing occupational niches to provide a more applied curriculum, and occupations aim to increase their social standing by obtaining university-level training to attain professional status.

In contrast to the dominant literature on the sociology of the professions, in which the drive for professionalisation is a struggle between established occupational groups to achieve social closure, the occupations described earlier have achieved professional status within a relatively consensual environment. There is no evidence of medical control or intervention into the scopes of practice of any of these professions, other than supporting the initial introduction of the ODP.

There is a need for closer examination of the regulatory and organisational frameworks in which new professions evolve. The centralised NHS model can place levers over workforce supply and demand that are not available in a more open-market environment such as the Australian health system. Conversely, the increasing drive for the professionalisation of the workforce may enhance quality and standards but the price is an increasing cost of providing healthcare.

FIVE

The support workforce within the allied health division of labour

This chapter examines the support workforce associated with the allied health professions. We have used the term 'support workers' to describe this group because they do not occupy a fully professional space, and they have emerged from the division of allied health labour (Saks and Allsop, 2007; Saks, 2020). We acknowledge that numerous other titles are used to describe workers in this domain of work (Buchan and Dal Poz, 2002; Saks and Allsop, 2007; Bach et al, 2008; Lizarondo et al, 2010). Support workers tend to be vocationally trained and, in many cases, their roles are designed and adapted to meet local requirements.

We distinguish the support workforce from the emerging and existing allied health professions on the basis that support worker roles are derived from the division of labour of existing allied health roles, whereas emerging professions (described in Chapter 4) have generally developed a niche professional repertoire and practise autonomously. Support workers are differentiated from 'professions' because they do not have ownership over a unique body of knowledge or theoretical framework that defines their role. Contemporary taxonomies of allied health professions tend to reinforce the notion of the professional project (Larson, 1977) by specifying minimum standards, such as required levels of training, continuing professional development, codes of conduct and quality monitoring standards (Health Care Professions Council, no date; Allied Health Aotearoa New Zealand, no date; Allied Health Professions Australia, no date). As we discuss in this chapter, there are few opportunities for support workers to become allied health professionals unless they meet these requirements.

The delegation of lower-status tasks to an auxiliary workforce is a well-established technique of professions to achieve internal closure (Hugman, 1991). However, the niche areas of practice and lack of recognised areas of specialisation have important implications for the roles of support workers and the advancement of the allied health professions. First, the clinical tasks that can be delegated by allied health professionals fall within a narrow scope of practice that is derived from the niche offering of the specific allied health profession. Second, allied health professions lack the internal professional career hierarchies that enable them to advance professionally as they cast off unwanted tasks to auxiliary staff within their own division of labour, losing some of the advantages of delegation that are apparent within the large professional hierarchies of medicine and nursing.

As highlighted in Chapter 1, contrary to the dominant, neo-Weberian sociology of the professions, in which professional groups discard unwanted tasks to free them up to perform more highly specialised roles, few allied health professions recognise endorsed specialities. Thus, in delegating clinical tasks, they inevitably become more involved in management or organisational tasks (McClimens et al, 2010). Lack of regulation of most allied health tasks means that there are few (if any) limitations to their transfer or delegation, which challenges the modern notion of the professional project which proposes that professions are actively attempting to protect their professional boundaries to maintain ownership over a discrete body of knowledge in order to sustain specific economic and status advantages. Indeed, it appears that the most significant drivers for the introduction of new support worker roles arose during the early 2000s, a time of substantial workforce shortages and rapid expansion of the NHS when there were some upward opportunities for allied health expansion (Aiken et al, 2008; Skinner et al, 2015). Later, in Australia, there were suggestions of impending workforce shortages, for which an assistant workforce was subsequently introduced as a solution (Duckett, 2005).

Perhaps as a result of the timing of and drivers for the introduction of the support worker roles, their rapid growth in the 2000s met with little opposition due to shortages of, and commensurate opportunities for expansion of, the other health professions. They are now an established workforce in many jurisdictions. There is some evidence of protectionary behaviour in the development of support roles but this has largely dissolved over the past few decades as the concept of auxiliary workers has become more acceptable.

The heterogeneity of the allied health professions means that their associated support workers will have even more diverse and complex considerations. Rather than attempt to address issues that are specific to every possible allied health discipline, this chapter will draw on the published accounts of the support worker roles associated with the allied health disciplines and attempt to draw out the issues and themes that are common across jurisdictions and professions.

The growth of support workers in allied health

Auxiliaries have probably existed in some form for as long as the professions. Allied health support workers were documented as early as the 1950s in occupational therapy in Canada (Salvatori, 2001) and, later, in physiotherapy and podiatry in the NHS in the UK (Webb et al, 2004). Allied health support workers were primarily introduced to increase the capacity of already stretched allied health professions and to allow existing practitioners to focus on more highly skilled areas of practice, while delegating unwanted or more routine tasks (Salvatori, 2001; Webb et al, 2004; Le Cornu et al, 2010). The interest in this workforce has increased under a managerial agenda that explores opportunities for efficiencies while reorienting care around more patient-centred principles (Nancarrow, 2020).

The allied health support workforce has evolved through two distinct models (Nancarrow, 2020). The first is the profession-driven model, which involves the delegation of roles to auxiliaries under the direction of allied health professionals. The second is the managerial model, which became increasingly dominant during the late 20th and early 21st centuries, resulting from large-scale workforce reform that created centralised support and development for support worker roles across a range of settings and jurisdictions. This has been supported by a suite of tools that has re-engineered the workforce around patient needs and risk, rather than professional preferences (Smith and Duffy, 2010; State of Victoria Department of Health and Human Services, 2016).

The managerial and professional agendas are not entirely independent. In some cases, the managerial agenda has supported the professional goals of growth of the allied health professions (Webb et al, 2004). Both approaches involve the codification and devolution of tasks from qualified allied health practitioners to auxiliaries, even if each approach has a different goal and the results are different.

The profession-driven model has focused on increasing the capacity of allied health professions under the division of labour of a single profession, primarily through the delegation of unwanted tasks under the direct supervision of an allied health professional. This provides increased opportunities for professionals to focus on more highly skilled and generally less technical tasks, and to increase the volume of patients seen.

Where the profession-driven model has been led by the professions, the managerial agenda has placed the responsibility for role renegotiation under the control of bureaucracies (Dent et al, 2004; State of Victoria

Department of Health and Human Services, 2016). Managerial drivers are bureaucratically inspired and more patient-focused, and increase the likelihood of delegating tasks from specific professions within a generic model of working. These approaches are explored more fully in this chapter.

The allied health division of labour

Increasingly, managerialism is seeing the reorganisation of work based on competence rather than professions (Nancarrow and Borthwick, 2005). In support of this, there is a growing tendency within the health professions, and particularly the allied health professions, to codify and commodify discrete tasks into 'competencies'. These competencies are then made available to other groups, either through horizontal task transfer (such as the allied health rural generalist pathway in Australia discussed in Chapter 7) or through the creation of a micro-specialism, in which high-volume, specialised tasks become the primary function of a niche technical group (such as cast technicians and newborn hearing-screening specialists).

Task-based allocation of work was proposed within the industrial notions of Taylorism in the late 19th and early 20th centuries (Littler, 1978; Berwick, 2003). Taylorism involves the analysis, breaking down and reallocation of tasks to the least-skilled, lowest-price worker eligible to deliver highly specialised tasks or skills. Health was slow to shift to a technically based framework. Instead, healthcare was strongly bound in sociopolitical negotiations about roles and tasks, and the inability to codify much of that work limited the transferability of tasks.

Later, in 1970, Jamous and Peloille (1970) proposed that professional work could be defined by a high proportion of tacit knowledge and expertise that was specific to that profession, which they termed indeterminacy. In contrast, less professional work was described as having a higher technical component. This became known as the 'technicality to indeterminacy ratio'. They, and others, argued that if professional groups codified their activities in terms of explicit practices and procedures, they risked losing control over those aspects of their work. Consequently, professions emphasised the indeterminacy components of their roles, which called for, and reinforced, the importance of their professional judgement.

However, several factors converged during the 20th century that resulted in allied health professions promoting the technicality of their roles. Scientific advances, alongside the growth of managerialism, increased the drive for the transparency and accountability of the health professions (Traynor, 2009). Several strategies were used to increase the reproducibility and codification of health professional work, including standardised higher education, evidence-based medicine, professional accreditation programmes and clinical guidelines.

As relatively new professions, the allied health professions were simultaneously involved in the act of demonstrating their effectiveness through research and evidence-based practice, while increasingly codifying their practice through competency-based training. Competencies have been embraced to such an extent that dedicated tools were developed specifically to systematically analyse allied health work and devolve professional roles into discrete tasks that could be codified into competencies. One of the first of these tools was the Calderdale Framework (Smith and Duffy, 2010). This framework has been adapted by other health organisations. For example, the Victorian Department of Health and Human Services has developed the Victorian Assistant Workforce Model (VAWM), which enables a systematic approach for the identification and quantification of work that can be delegated from allied health professionals to allied health assistants (State of Victoria Department of Health and Human Services, 2016; Somerville et al, 2018).

Other recent innovations that support the codification of work practices are the growth of microcredentialing and micro-specialisms. Micro-specialisms are high-volume and generally low-risk tasks that have normally developed from the division of labour of an established role. They tend to involve a short training time to learn a particular task to meet a specific, focused need. Examples that could be classified as micro-specialisms include newborn hearing screening, phlebotomy, cast technicians, foot care assistants and the reduction of some of the core components of acupuncture to dry needling (Nancarrow, 2015; Zhou et al, 2015).

Microcredentialing is a relatively new technology to verify activities that do not require the level of endorsement of a full qualification (such as a degree or diploma). Instead, microcredentials enable a credentialing body or training provider to establish the necessary criteria to demonstrate that specific skills or competencies have been achieved. Microcredentials can be delivered using a range of flexible approaches, including online, in the workplace or at a training institution. They tend to be shorter than traditional degrees and certificates (Cathrael Kazin and Clerkin, 2018). Microcredentials can be delivered by a range of providers, though it is likely that the credibility of the training provider will be an important component of their trustworthiness. There is also the potential to 'bundle' microcredentials together to build a portfolio of evidence that can count towards formal certification or qualifications.

At the time of writing, the use of microcredentials in healthcare is not widespread. However, the allied health professions have strongly embraced the codification and commodification of competencies in healthcare delivery. The microcredentialing approach will support this approach, and potentially disrupt the way that the health workforce is trained.

This chapter explores two case studies of allied health support workers. The first is the introduction of an OTA practitioner in North Staffordshire in 2004. The second is the introduction of a podiatry assistant in the ACT in 2012. We have used these examples because they were both relatively new innovations at the time of development, and both have detailed contextual data available. These examples juxtapose the introduction of support worker roles in Australia and the UK, in a highly technical role (podiatry assistant) versus, arguably, a less technical role (OTA).

Occupational therapy assistant practitioners

Occupational therapy is a client-centred health profession concerned with promoting health and well-being through engagement in daily occupations. The primary goal of occupational therapy is to enable people to participate in the activities of everyday life. Occupational therapists achieve this outcome by working with people and communities to enhance their ability to engage in the occupations they want to, need to or are expected to, or by modifying the occupation or the environment to better support their occupational engagement (World Federation of Occupational Therapists, 2012). Occupational therapists are registered with the HCPC in the UK and with the Australian Health Practitioner Regulation Agency (AHPRA) in Australia.

Occupational therapy support workers have a long history of assisting occupational therapists in administrative and housekeeping tasks, as well as during the therapy process, including programme planning, intervention and evaluation. The question of roles and boundaries between qualified occupational therapists and their support workers has been debated intermittently in the international literature on occupational therapy (Atkinson, 1993; Hirama, 1994; Von Zweck, 1998; Salvatori, 2001).

In the UK, the College of Occupational Therapists (COT) first endorsed the role of an occupational therapy support worker in 1993

(College of Occupational Therapists, 1993). Support workers were introduced to address chronic workforce shortages and also respond to increasing managerial demands to use support staff more effectively (Atkinson, 1993). Originally, the COT proposed that the initial assessment of all those referred should be carried out by a qualified occupational therapist but that certain aspects of a more comprehensive assessment may be carried out by trained support workers. Towards the end of the 1990s, increasing demand for occupational therapy services and the continuing shortfall in the numbers of qualified therapists led to advocates for an extended role for occupational therapy support workers that included an assessment role.

At the end of the 20th century, several factors converged in the UK that resulted in a renewed focus on the health workforce. These included the introduction of the European Working Time Directive, as well as increasing pressures on the workforce from an ageing population. There were multiple policy responses from around 2000 that explicitly drove workforce modernisation and change. These included the NHS human resources strategy, *HR in the NHS Plan* (Department of Health, 2002). The key themes involve a strategy for growing and developing the NHS workforce, a major redesign of jobs, the introduction of a 'skills escalator' to promote career progression and personal development, and a fair pay system that would reward staff according to the value of their work, rather than to hierarchical and complex pay scales (Skills for Health, no date). The Changing Workforce Programme (CWP) was established within the NHS Modernisation Agency to promote the development of new and extended roles. The introduction of support workers and 'assistant practitioners', who are higher-level support workers that complement the work of registered professionals, was one of the modernisation initiatives promoted by the CWP (Changing Workforce Programme, 2003). The CWP recommended that support workers should have access to nationally recognised qualifications and, as such, many forms of vocational qualifications were developed, including foundation degrees and updated National Vocational Qualifications (NVQs).

This rapidly evolving practice environment required occupational therapists to examine their own roles, boundaries and relationships. North Staffordshire Combined Healthcare Trust responded by introducing seven new OTA practitioner posts based at the primary and secondary care interface. The therapy assistant practitioner was an extension of the existing OTA role. The following case study draws on data from an evaluation of the introduction of that role (Mackey and Nancarrow, 2004, 2005; Nancarrow and Borthwick, 2005).

Within North Staffordshire, OTA practitioners are defined as practitioners who: can work autonomously on an occupational therapy caseload; can assess occupational therapy need and deliver occupational therapy interventions but 'know their own boundaries and capabilities and will not exceed those' (Mackey and Nancarrow, 2004: 4); are supervised by a qualified occupational therapist but responsible for the outcomes of their own patients; have a vocational qualification; and can deliver occupational therapy and 'generic' roles without direct supervision in a range of health and social care settings. The roles and responsibilities of the OTA were determined by a local working party that established the work procedures, job descriptions and a definition of the OTA, which was that the OTA is 'a support worker who, through extra training, is able to practise autonomously, make decisions, and instigate treatment based on those decisions and is accountable for his or her own practice' (Mackey and Nancarrow, 2004: 13).

The OTA introduction coincided with the implementation of Agenda for Change in the UK. Agenda for Change introduced a common grading system across all nursing and allied health workers (Department of Health, 2004b). The roles were established using the previous (Whitley Council Technical Instructor) scale but were benchmarked as equivalent to an Agenda for Change Band 4 (below professional level). Eligibility to apply to be an OTA required two years' relevant experience in health or social care and a relevant (level 3) qualification. The position was developed with a view to clinicians being eligible for promotion to an Agenda for Change Band 5 on completion of the vocational training and a review of roles and responsibilities.

The OTAs worked autonomously. In exploring the differentiation between the OTA and the occupational therapist, both groups of practitioners perceived that the OTAs could perform most of the roles undertaken by the qualified occupational therapists except for home visits. Negotiating the boundaries of what the OTA could and could not do proved challenging. For example, OTAs were able to assist occupational therapists with pre-discharge visits but were not allowed to perform home visits on their own. In some cases, the only time the qualified occupational therapist would see the patient was at the home visit, with the OTA having delivered all prior care. This created gaps in continuity and consistency of care for the patient and the practitioner.

There was a suggestion that the qualified occupational therapist would see the more 'complex' cases but no one could define what complex meant in this context. It was unclear whether complexity referred to the clinical diagnoses or social complexity. This model was further challenged because if a qualified occupational therapist was not available to treat a complex case, the OTA would fill the role. Similarly, OTAs reported that when the occupational therapist was present, their scope of practice reduced because much of their work was undertaken by the occupational therapist. As the OTAs highlighted, if they are deemed competent to work to a specific scope of practice, then they should be enabled and, indeed, expected to consistently work to this level.

A key differentiator between the OTA tasks and those of the occupational therapist was described as the emphasis by the occupational therapists on the theory and philosophy of occupation. In other words, occupational therapy expertise or indeterminacy was symbolised by the theory of occupation. One OTA described this in the following way: 'we have got the brickwork, we have got the foundations and it is just putting in the bits in between really. It is your [the OT] understanding of why you do things this way and what is behind it' (Mackey and Nancarrow, 2004: 22). The delineation of roles was further complicated because the occupational therapists reported that their role had shifted from a focus on occupation to the delivery of tasks. This was articulated well by the following occupational therapist:

> We've suddenly developed dressing practices in OT [occupational therapy] role, transfer practice, and actually we've lost the occupational meaning behind those roles, so suddenly this is a task. So we end up now in this new position of trying to defend tasks when really we shouldn't be taking a task approach, it's what we bring as professionals with their own background about the essence. (Mackey and Nancarrow, 2004: 23)

This supports the idea that clinical expertise, or the indeterminacy of roles, becomes devalued or lost in a system that values technical expertise (Copnell, 2010).

Career development of the OTAs followed a professional, not a managerial path, with those OTAs who wanted to progress undertaking training to become a qualified occupational therapist, despite managerial options being available within the service. The professional (clinical) pathway was perceived by OTAs as being of higher status than the managerial path. In contrast, the only progression opportunity available for occupational therapists in this setting was management. Interestingly, there were suggestions that the qualified occupational therapists did not want to delegate to OTAs because they would lose the job satisfaction associated with treating patients. In other words, the delegation of technical tasks to OTAs eroded the technical skills of the occupational therapists. The managerial agenda of the NHS did not value their expertise or their philosophy of practice, leaving the occupational therapists with a management pathway if they wanted to progress.

One suggestion was that despite most of the delegated tasks being technical tasks, occupational therapists perceived that there might be an opportunity to delegate management tasks to OTAs in order to free them up to perform more clinical tasks. This reflected a preference of the occupational therapists to perform clinical rather than management roles. The introduction of the OTA was not seen to support the specialisation of occupational therapists, and the qualified occupational therapists reported that they were losing what they called 'specialised skills', such as splinting, at the risk of becoming more generic.

The way that the OTA interacted with the patients differed to that of the qualified occupational therapists. For instance, OTAs spent more time with the patients than the qualified occupational therapists, and therefore perceived that they had a better understanding of the patient and their needs. Patients were unconcerned about the training or professional status of the staff member, but valued having increased time with the staff. Similarly, the OTAs came from the local community and, as a result, there were suggestions that they could more closely identify with the patients' needs 'because they are from a similar background to the clients and do not use complicated language' (Mackey and Nancarrow, 2004: 25).

However, within the occupational therapy service, managers recognised that class and language barriers between qualified and unqualified staff could enhance the relationships between assistant practitioners and users as the support workers were representatives of the communities they served, rather than those of the professions. The role of language in asserting professional power and occupational hierarchies is well documented (Saks, 2016).

The status of professions has long been linked with that of their associates and patients or clients (Leicht and Fennell, 2001). Indeed, the dominance of the medical profession was initially enhanced by the elevated position of their patients. Similarly, the early development of physiotherapy received royal patronage and was linked to well-to-do clients, which substantially increased the standing of the profession (Larkin, 1983). However, with support workers, the converse may be true. In this example, OTA practitioner roles were developed, in part, to provide work for local factory hands following the closure of the potteries in Staffordshire (Nancarrow and Mackey, 2005).

However, their class background and a lack of university education meant that assistant practitioners 'spoke a different language' to qualified occupational therapists and were more closely aligned with their patients.

The managerial agenda could be seen to be forcibly undermining class agendas by shifting healthcare delivery from powerful elites to auxiliaries and laypeople, and even the lay workforce. The healthcare division of labour is also heavily influenced within the managerial model by different perspectives on types of illness and associated healthcare activities. To a certain extent, the class divisions between the OTA and the occupational therapist are a reflection of Marxist theories and the role and dominance of the 'middle-class professional' (Navarro, 1978; Doyal, 1979). However, interestingly in this case, rather than the OTA accruing power by associating with middle-class clients, they are achieving a relative benefit in their relationship to the patient because they are not middle class. The OTAs are better able to relate to the clients they work with. This provides the OTAs with a relative therapeutic benefit over the qualified occupational therapists because they spend more time with the client, and have a better understanding of, and relationships within, the local context.

Supervision and accountability were key areas for discussion around the implementation of the OTA role. Formal and informal supervision structures were established for the OTA. Formal supervision needed to be regular and with an identified member of staff. The purpose of the supervision was to ensure the competence of the OTA, provide pastoral support and support the clinical role. Informal supervision provided the opportunity for the OTA to address immediate and important clinical concerns with any member of staff. However, a challenge of the supervisory relationships was the lack of training provided to the qualified occupational therapists to supervise support staff.

A further point of ambiguity was the accountability for the outcomes of the care. In particular, there was a lack of clarity around who was responsible for the outcomes of care if it was delegated to an OTA. There was an assumption that if the care was delegated to an OTA, that the delegating occupational therapist would be responsible for the outcome of that care. This is a concern that has arisen in other contexts (Timmons and Tanner, 2004) and can result in an unwillingness to delegate.

The lack of a regulatory framework for the OTA was a further point of confusion. Despite the occupational therapist and the OTA performing almost indistinguishable tasks, there were no restrictions on the practice of the OTA. In contrast, an occupational therapist who had not paid their registration fee was unable to practise as an occupational therapist, even though the tasks are similar. This calls into question the value of a regulation framework that enables less-skilled workers to perform the same tasks purely on the basis of a bureaucratic formality.

Related to the issues of accountability and responsibility was the determination of competence of an OTA. The completion of a vocational qualification was seen to provide a level of implied responsibility, even though many of the courses were not directly relevant to the OTA role. The lack of trust in the new roles was partly associated with it being a new role. This resulted in a high level of mistrust from the qualified occupational therapists, who had not had a direct role in the oversight and development of the new OTA role.

Formal training involved the use of some 'off the shelf' vocational qualifications that, at that stage, had not been tailored to the OTA role because it was new. As a result, the qualification was seen to have peripheral relevance to the actual practice of the OTA role. The occupational therapists valued on-the-job training and the development of experience; however, the formal qualification was seen as an important process of verification for ensuring clinical governance. A lack of understanding of the structure and content of the vocational qualifications led to some qualified occupational therapists dismissing them as a token form of formal verification of competence (Mackey and Nancarrow, 2005), a factor that has been found elsewhere (Hancock et al, 2005).

Several key issues exist around the role boundaries between support workers and allied health professionals. The modern health workforce typically requires qualified, autonomous health practitioners to have control over a body of work. This model is based on a structure where those at the top of the hierarchy determine the division of labour by creating rules that dictate what roles can be given away to other workers and formal boundaries to protect their own roles (Hugman, 1991). A great deal of energy in health workforce reform is based on determining what can be delegated to whom. However, as this study shows, there is evidence that, in many cases, supervising practitioners do not delegate consistently or to the full extent of the scope of practice of the delegate, resulting in inefficiencies in the use of the delegate.

This study identifies two broad categories for failure to delegate effectively, namely: (1) regulatory or accountability barriers to delegation; and (2) discretionary delegation. The regulatory/accountability barriers to delegation arise from a lack of clear accountability structures or regulation of the tasks, which prevents delegation. Discretionary delegation arises when the delegating practitioner: is uncertain of the skills of the person to whom they are delegating; wants to retain their own workload; lacks confidence in the delegate because of the mistrust or inexperience of the delegating practitioner; lacks the skills to delegate; lacks an understanding of role boundaries or perceives a threat to professionalism; or does not value the potential of delegation.

Workforce efficiency is optimised when the workplace environment enables staff to work to their full scope of practice. Inefficient delegation arises when practitioners practise 'discretionary' delegation, that is, the delegating practitioner effectively determines the scope of practice of the delegate in situ.

Podiatry assistants

Podiatrists are primary healthcare practitioners of the feet and lower limb. Podiatrists provide assessment, advice and treatment for skin and nail conditions of the feet, provide footwear advice and modification, manage foot complications associated with diabetes, and perform surgical treatment of ingrown toenails.

This discussion focuses on the introduction of podiatry assistants in Australia and the UK, where there is a limited documented history and relatively similar background (Webb et al, 2004). Podiatry assistants were first formally introduced in response to podiatry workforce shortages in England by the NHS in 1977, initially as foot hygienists under the supervision of podiatrists (Webb et al, 2004). The introduction of foot hygienists met with mixed responses from the profession and the wider community. Age Concern, an organisation representing the views of older people, perceived that the shortage of podiatry services reflected a lack of prioritisation by the state of foot care services for older people. Conversely, a member of the profession suggested that this was a good opportunity for stratification of, and specialisation within, the profession to meet sociopolitical pressure and to facilitate professional expansion. The Chiropodists Board (as it was known at the time) was resistant to the concept of auxiliary grades within the profession because of concerns they might compete with podiatrists working in the private sector, patients being put at risk and the protection of the professional status of podiatrists:

> Many members will still hold feelings of strong aversion to the training of footcare assistants … the thought of people doing an 'easy' course of study has become increasingly obnoxious to those successfully completing the only course of study leading to eligibility for membership of

the Society of Chiropodists and state registration. This anathema has been exacerbated by numerous stories of footcare assistants who, having built up a level of dexterity, have set themselves up as 'chiropodist' in the private sector. (Editorial, 1989: 265)

The government was supportive of the development of auxiliaries due to the perceived potential for cost savings in service delivery. Despite these varying perspectives, the assistant role was introduced.

Following introduction of the role, training for the assistants became a point of contention. Initially, it was felt that a formal training structure was unnecessary due to the relatively basic nature of the delegated tasks, and that those tasks would be performed under supervision. Additionally, the development of more formal training met with resistance from the profession on the basis that codification of practice for auxiliaries would further increase the risk of competition to the profession in an unregulated sector. Professional bodies representing podiatrists across the UK felt that the scope of practice for the assistant role should be limited to activities that a normal healthy adult would be able to perform for themselves.

Instead of introducing formal training, the early scope of the podiatry assistant role was determined by case-by-case delegation from the supervising podiatrist. However, it quickly became apparent that this model was creating large disparities in the way the podiatry assistant role was being implemented. Consequently, the Association of Chief Chiropody Officers introduced a six-month vocational training programme that included a final exam. Several podiatry departments adopted this training programme. At the time, there was some discussion about incorporating the assistant training into the podiatry school training pathway. While NHS managers supported the training pathway approach, ultimately, local training was perceived to better meet local requirements, and was cheaper to deliver.

Supervision of the role was a further consideration. Initially, podiatrists could only employ assistants if they directly supervised those assistants. Direct supervision was defined as the podiatrist being present in the same room as the assistant performing treatment. There were suggestions that if this level of supervision was not adhered to, the podiatrist would be liable in the event of a claim of adverse outcomes of the treatment delivered by the assistant. The inefficiencies associated with implementing this level of supervision meant that further development of the podiatry assistant role ceased until clear boundaries between the roles of the podiatrist and the assistant were determined. Such proximal supervision is not feasible or practical, and the role has been continued under a more devolved level of supervision. However, the College of Podiatry (2020) specifies that while the assistant practitioner is accountable to an HCPC registered podiatrist and works under the direct supervision of a podiatrist, the two do not need to be co-located, and that delegation should be in line with the skills and competence of the podiatry assistant.

The scope of practice of podiatry assistants initially involved cutting toenails and preparing patients for foot surgery. While few other areas of scope were made explicit, the point of demarcation for podiatrists and assistants appeared to be the use of a scalpel for tissue debridement (primarily the removal of corns and callus).

The UK College of Podiatry now recognises a suite of 'assistant practitioners' in the field of podiatry, which include foot care assistants, orthotic technicians and podiatry assistants. The college specifies that the role will be locally determined by the employing organisation but that the scope must not exceed the guidelines published by the college, which excludes debridement with a scalpel. The scope is broadly defined as: administrative tasks, such as information management, communication, record keeping, research data collection and stock control; clinical skills, such as patient and clinic preparation, and application of skin care products; administering a physical therapy or wound management care plan; managing pathological nails on low-risk patients; and miscellaneous duties, such as health education and diabetes screening. The types of patients that assistants are able to see are 'low-risk' patients or those with low or no medical or podiatric need.

In 2002, podiatry assistants were granted associate membership of the College of Podiatry following a model that was introduced by the Chartered Society of Physiotherapy some time earlier. Membership provides assistants with access to professional networks, newsletters and trade union and employment support.

Another analysis of the employment of foot care assistants in the UK (Farndon and Nancarrow, 2003) found that some podiatry services did not employ foot care assistants because the health service prioritised 'high-risk' care at the expense of 'low-risk' podiatry work. So-called 'low-risk' care, which included basic foot care and nail maintenance, was not seen to be the remit of the health service. The use of foot care assistants was seen to increase the opportunities for podiatrists to specialise. However, none of the 'specialisations' identified were formally recognised and most were extensions of the existing scope of practice of podiatrists. Instead, the use of foot care assistants enabled podiatrists in larger departments to concentrate on niche areas of interest, while delegating, or ignoring, the low-status, low-risk tasks. The risk of this approach was that podiatrists lost ownership of the so-called 'low-risk' tasks, potentially to other untrained or unskilled practitioners.

As with the UK, the establishment of podiatry assistants in Australia met with mixed responses from the profession. The issues that faced podiatry assistants are reminiscent of the tensions created by the early introduction of most allied health support worker roles. These focused on resisting threats to the monopolies of the allied professions through boundary maintenance and the creation of status hierarchies through the development of subordinate grades subject to the control of professionals (Larkin, 1983; Webb et al, 2004). Opponents to allied health support workers have expressed concerns that the introduction of support workers is merely a way to provide allied healthcare at a lower cost, leading to deprofessionalisation (Braverman, 1974; Webb et al, 2004; Le Cornu et al, 2010). In Australia, the public–private and state–federal fragmentation of healthcare means that there are jurisdictional variations in the introduction of allied health support workers, and much of this is poorly documented.

One study on the introduction of podiatry assistants from the ACT found that a shortage of podiatry services was being addressed by the delegation of basic foot care services to enrolled nurses managed under the nursing division of labour (Moran et al, 2012). This meant that podiatrists lost ownership over a component of their core business to the larger group of nurses, and their patients were managed under the nursing, not podiatry, team. This created a disjointed service pathway and clinical governance concerns about foot care services – as well as unhappiness among some enrolled nurses about being delegated the low-status, discarded foot care role.

In response, the ACT government Health Service Directorate introduced the podiatry assistant role to help meet patient needs and to improve the quality of the patient experience by integrating podiatric care under the podiatry division of labour. The role was also designed to reduce workforce shortages, and to enable the podiatrists to see the 'high-risk' patients and leave the 'low-risk' care to the assistants. The risk status of the client was determined by an initial assessment performed by the podiatrists, who would then allocate the most appropriate provider of care based on that risk assessment.

In the Australian study, there was a clear delineation between the work that a podiatry assistant could perform and that of a qualified podiatrist (Moran et al, 2012). One task – the use of a scalpel – was restricted by ACT legislation at the time the role was being developed, with the (then) ACT Podiatrist's Board stating that restricted duties include treatment involving the use of a scalpel. Having clearly defined competencies provided reassurance to both the podiatry assistants about their scope of work and the podiatrists. This was important because, as with the OTA study earlier, the podiatrists expressed concern about accountability for the outcomes of the care of the podiatry assistants.

Both podiatry examples demonstrate how podiatrists lost professional control of a component of their work during a time of workforce shortages. In Australia, the service was delivered outside the supervision of podiatrists as they surrendered their division of labour to nurses – illustrating the importance of either employing auxiliaries within the division of labour of the allied health practitioners or the risk of losing control over that domain of work. The podiatrists in this example were able to regain control over their core business through the reallocation of roles to newly developed support workers because nurses and podiatrists were employed within the same community organisation. However, had the enrolled nurses been employed separately, it is possible that the roles would not have been returned. Interestingly, the introduction of the podiatry assistant did not impact the workload of podiatrists because it only resulted in the transfer of foot care work previously performed by enrolled nurses. In the UK, low-risk foot care was deemed by podiatrists to be of sufficiently low priority and status to completely disregard this work. The services that employed podiatry assistants maintained such foot care within their division of labour; however, other services effectively dropped this low-risk, low-status work from their repertoire to focus on higher-risk and higher-status 'virtuoso' roles such as diabetes management and biomechanics (Hugman, 1991). This was despite the concerns from private podiatrists that unregulated practitioners would step in and take over basic foot care.

A more recent example of an allied health support worker is the dietetic support worker introduced by the British Dietetics Association to reduce the increasing incidence of malnutrition among hospital in-patients. This role was led by the profession, drawing on successful models of support worker implementation from the US. It reflected the changing sociopolitical landscape in following the introduction of the evidence-based medicine movement and in responding to perceived service needs, including efficiency and patient-centred values, supported by the managerial agenda (Le Cornu et al, 2010). The role of the dietetic support worker therefore met with little professional resistance as it fell within tightly constrained boundaries under the supervisory control of the dietetics profession.

Discussion

The case studies presented in this chapter illustrate an interesting challenge for allied health. On the one hand, managerialism combined with workforce shortages is forcing the allied health professions to deconstruct their technical roles into codifiable, commodifiable tasks. These competencies can potentially be performed by anyone with the appropriate skills and training. Simultaneously, the indeterminacy components of allied health roles are being eroded or ignored by funding and commissioning pressures that instead focus on the delivery of tasks rather than the core philosophies of the profession.

The ultimate extrapolation of this process is that allied health roles become eroded into a suite of disconnected tasks that can be reconstructed and reconfigured into new functions that meet the needs of the end user or purchaser of the services. The question that needs to be asked is whether these disembodied tasks actually require the organising and philosophical frame of a profession, or they can be safely and adequately delivered out of their professional context. The answer probably lies in the context and application of those tasks. In some instances, such as those illustrated in these case studies, the disaggregation of tasks is entirely appropriate. In others, the organising frame of the profession will be required. Wilensky (1964) used the metaphor of an engineer and a technician involved in building a bridge. He proposed that, ultimately, all labour is rooted in theory, and supported this by proposing that while the civil engineer who designs a bridge may know some laws of physics, the workers who build the bridge do not. In other words, there is a need for a unifying expertise or philosophy that provides a guiding framework for the technical roles. It appears that the unifying expertise in these examples may not be technical, but managerial. This concept is revisited again in Chapter 7 in the case of the rural generalist allied health practitioner, where the technical roles are deconstructed but there is an assumption of a 'core' of managerial expertise. The extrapolation of this model is that allied health practitioners would delegate all their technical roles and instead maintain a managerial relationship with the health system and the patient. This may be a model of healthcare brokering based on diagnoses and or assessment of patient needs, signposting and guiding patients to appropriate services in a complex system.

The introduction of allied health support workers is largely driven by a need to address workforce shortages. It is unclear what will happen to the support roles if the shortages of the core professions are resolved. As Abbott (1988) suggests, professions can not only gain privileges through jurisdictional work claims, but, as the example of the OTA shows, also easily lose privileges too. Managerial drivers are unlikely to support the unwinding of a lower-cost workforce, yet there are not sufficient advancement opportunities for the allied health professions to continue to pursue an upward professional trajectory.

In contrast to Hughes's notion of 'ditching the dirty work' (Hugman, 1991), it seems that the delegated tasks are often integral to the identity of the professionals. The occupational therapists, particularly, resisted the notion of giving away components of their work because it was those components that gave their roles meaning. It is also interesting that both podiatrists and occupational therapists are state-registered professions in both Australia and the UK. Yet, both professions have the potential to delegate a very large proportion of their work to an unregulated workforce under a managerial agenda that largely protects the patients through organisational clinical governance, not state regulation. This brings into question the value of state regulation of the professions as a tool for protecting the public. Only one task was restricted in this case: the use of a scalpel by podiatry assistants.

A further important driver here is the increasingly complex needs of patients and the contexts in which care is provided. As patient care and patient needs move outside the structures of formal occupational or organisational hierarchy – such as a hospital – into complex care environments and complex needs, it makes sense that roles and tasks need to be reconfigured to more appropriately meet those needs. This reflects Noordegraaf's (2007) transition from pure to hybrid professionalism. Noordegraaf describes a shift from a formal, traditional, pure or 'occupational profession', which is based on technical rationality and focused on solving specific problems for certain cases (clients), to an 'organisational profession'. His 'organisational profession' was largely embedded in public service roles that traditionally do not hold professional status. In the case of the allied health professions, we are seeing a transition to a model of managerial professionalism that is based on the assessment, organisation and allocation of tasks around the needs of patients. They may be guided by an occupational philosophy (such as the philosophy of occupation, as in occupational therapy) or by the framework of the organisation (such as a disability service). Shifting care away from the organisational hierarchy of the hospital into the community or patients' own homes provides a radical departure from the traditional institutionally bound divisions of labour, control of technology and determination of roles (Turner, 1995; Zagrodney and Saks, 2017).

The challenge for the allied health professions is that their training lures them into a unidisciplinary, professionally focused model of healthcare delivery. In some settings, that model will remain, but as healthcare becomes increasingly complex, the more responsive approach is likely to increase. Indeed, several tools already exist facilitate the consensual reconfiguration of workforce roles (Smith and Duffy, 2010; State of Victoria Department of Health and Human Services, 2016; Pain et al, 2018). Additionally, professional status is associated with clinical specialisation, not with managerial responsibility. However, while this model presents a challenge for the allied health professions to respond to, it seems to present more appropriate, streamlined and continuous care for the patients.

Understanding the support workforce associated with allied health professions in Australia and the UK is complicated by the diversity of professions that are incorporated within the allied health umbrella and the range of contexts and jurisdictions in which they work. The roles are further confounded by the increasing influence of the state and bureaucracies on the development of the support worker role, shifting tasks from a clear discipline-specific division of labour to the ultimate 'boundary-spanning role': taking on tasks delegated from multiple professions; delivering care in a range of settings; and working across different employer and jurisdictional boundaries. This approach contrasts with the typically more unified, neo-Weberian focus on the professional project, in which groups establish common goals and tasks, as well as a common philosophy, to achieve monopolisation (Nancarrow and Borthwick, 2005; Saks, 2010, 2014).

SIX

Specialisation in allied health

There are several allied health professions that may be regarded as 'mature', in the sense that they have become an established part of mainstream health service provision, been recognised by the state and have a voice at policy level (Larkin, 1983; Hugman, 1991; Witz, 1992). Within that broad definition, they are also marked by a structure characterised by internal divisions recognised as specialisms within the discipline, demanding further forms of education, training and credentialing beyond baseline registration requirements (Hugman, 1991). Largely, these specialist fields of practice comprise roles with higher-level skills and knowledge, and thus attract a greater degree of prestige and, commonly, better remuneration (Hugman, 1991; Borthwick, 2000). While many of the long-standing allied health professions possess some types of internally recognised speciality forms of practice, relatively few enjoy state recognition in the guise of separate regulatory provisions or legislation. However, state health policies aimed at workforce flexibility have led to new opportunities for allied health professions to secure formal recognition for roles that were previously exclusive to the medical profession.

A discussion of the pursuit of specialisation for physiotherapists in Australia sheds light on some of the challenges faced by allied health professions as they seek to develop their own recognised specialisms (Bennett and Grant, 2004). In particular, the specialist areas need to be: recognised by peers and external agencies; associated with a career structure for clinicians; and associated with a commensurate remuneration and reward structure. Interestingly, the Physiotherapy Board of New Zealand (2020) endorses and regulates a range of specialisations within the physiotherapy profession, such as pelvic health, neurology, older adults, paediatrics and hand therapy. Other areas of practice may be endorsed at the discretion of the board. It is unclear whether, or how, they have addressed the issues raised by Bennet and Grant, and how these endorsed specialities differ in practice from special interests supported by other professional groups and bodies, with the exception of the endorsed, regulated title.

A growing area of expanded practice for allied health practitioners is the acquisition of legal rights to independently prescribe medicines; another is the legitimated practice of invasive surgery by non-medically qualified allied health professions. The profession of podiatry serves as a good example of a mature allied profession that has attained both (Borthwick, 2000; Borthwick et al, 2010, 2015).

How these allied health professions have attained formal recognition for their internal divisions, badged as 'specialisms', and why they have done so may be explained, in part, through the application of theory. There is little doubt that the profession of medicine may serve as an exemplar of a successful profession characterised by differing fields of specialism, each of which is assigned a different degree of professional status within the hierarchy of the profession itself (Leicht and Fennell, 2001). For Leicht and Fennell, medical specialisms that deal with stigmatised groups of patients, such as the elderly, infectious or mentally ill, fair less well in the hierarchy than the more prestigious fields that involve heroic interventions or highly technical procedures (such as cardiac surgery, paediatrics or neurosurgery). Zetka (2003, 2011) also explored the way in which an emergent specialism within medicine (obstetrics and gynaecology) fought for formal recognition, as well as space, within the hierarchy of esteem when adopting sophisticated technologies that disrupted the established hierarchies (notably, laparoscopy). Hugman (1991) outlined the way in which health professions operate a form of occupational closure internally, leading to the creation of new, higher-status 'virtuoso' roles at the upper end of the spectrum, incorporated as specialisms, while also identifying lower-level tasks that are then assigned to subordinate grades within the profession, such as aides or assistants.

Indeed, it has been suggested that internally developed 'specialisms' may be considered for analytic purposes as comparable to distinct professions as they also emerge, develop and are even superseded as a result of similar underpinning drivers (Pickard, 2010). Furthermore, professions subjected to exclusion by other, more powerful, professions attempt to distinguish themselves from it, while adopting their own exclusionary tactics, producing internal hierarchies of status (Macdonald, 1995).

In this respect, the allied health professions are templates against which the theory can be applied. Podiatric surgery is a useful exemplar of the dual strategies adopted by podiatrists. In seeking to specialise in a field that offers an elevated status beyond the profession's baseline practice, it sets its own boundaries of practice while avoiding amalgamation with, or absorption by, the more powerful competitor medical specialism (orthopaedic surgery). Doing so enables it to separate itself internally (within the profession) from general podiatry (often referred to as 'core' podiatry) (Farndon et al, 2006), using the mandate of advanced skills, higher-level credentials and state regulation.

Hugman's theoretical variant on closure, named 'internal closure', has resonance for the allied health professions, most clearly expressed in the regulated and structured internal divisions of the 'mature' allied health professions. It is worth dwelling on Hugman's model of 'internal closure', and his refinement of the notion of 'virtuoso' roles, as these hold the key to understanding the internal structure of a number of the allied health professions (as well as nursing). Hugman (1991), citing Howe (1986), uses the notion of 'ditching the dirty work' to describe the process of assigning lower-status tasks to subordinate workers, who are neither fully part of, nor clearly distinct from, the profession itself (such as 'aides' or 'assistant' grades). In adopting this manoeuvre, the allied health professions create space to allow themselves to lay claim to higher-status activities, usually based on theoretical knowledge (Hugman, 1991). By asserting a level of skill that matches the acquired knowledge, these professions seek to elevate their status through the adoption of increasingly complex 'specialist' roles, carrying greater risks and responsibilities than their 'generalist' counterparts. Essential to these roles is their 'glamour'; they are 'virtuoso' roles, reflecting enhanced skills, knowledge, autonomy and outcomes that are clearly measurable and quite specific, as well as being 'curing' rather than 'caring' (Davies, 1985). This latter point resonates with the literature on gender in the allied health professions (addressed in Chapter 2), and the exemplar here – podiatric surgery – typifies it as a male-dominated speciality.

For the allied health professions, the use of specialist knowledge and skills to elevate status has a particular relevance, for it allows a response to attempts at exclusion by more powerful professions that may dispute their knowledge base and claimed expertise. Equally, having identified and acquired these prestigious skills and forms of knowledge, those within the new 'specialism' seek to establish boundaries around themselves. They create and establish their own entry criteria, standard setting, assessment and governance, each designed to cleave the profession internally and restrict entry to a new elite. Hugman (1991) also noted a tendency among the professions' generalists to view their specialists as overqualified, and potentially as forming a new profession.

The distinction between nurses, midwives and health visitors is viewed in much the same way, and serves as a useful exemplar. Elaborating on the 'curing' versus 'caring' aspect of role status, Hugman echoes Leicht and Fennell's (2001) view of the importance of client type in determining whether roles constitute virtuoso specialist work or mundane, generalist fare. Work with children is seen as higher-status than work with elderly patients, and treatment of acute disorders is seen as more prestigious work than the management of chronic conditions

(Hugman, 1991: 99). One further facet of professionalisation that is identified by Hugman, and that arguably holds particular importance for the allied health professions, is captured in his maxim that 'The company by which you are judged includes colleagues as well as clients', implying that the relative status of the generalists outside the profession may act as a disadvantage to the ambitions of the specialists within it (Hugman, 1991: 101). In turn, the specialists might then seek to further distance themselves from their origins and become a new and separate professional group, requiring separate recognition through credentialism, regulation or legislation.

Freidson (1970, 1988), in his early work on the medical profession and its relationships with the other healthcare professions, pointed to the importance of higher-status roles in defining interprofessional power. By failing to secure a discrete area of work distinct from medicine and that can be practised without dependence on, or the involvement of, medicine, the non-medical professions were doomed to subordination. For Freidson (1988), the power of medicine to subordinate the allied health professions (paramedical professions, in his parlance) centred on its absolute control of the central elements of diagnosis, surgery and prescribing, as the paramedical professions' work formed a penumbra around it, and was thus dependent upon it. If we now use these three key roles as an exemplar, and explore the ways in which allied health professions have sought to challenge medical exclusivity in these areas, it becomes possible to examine the extent of change in allied health professional power. This enables us to focus on the interprofessional conflict that has resulted from a challenge to medicine's core functions and roles, as distinct from more peripheral, less contested roles.

Clearly, the struggle for professionalism by those allied health professions, ranged against the weight of medical resistance, highlights the ongoing relevance of neo-Weberian explanations (King et al, 2015; King, 2018). However, it is also important to add a note of caution in the application of some aspects of some earlier neo-Weberian assumptions, particularly in relation to specialist technical expertise. Recent authors have stressed the gradual erosion of professional power and loss of autonomy through codification, such as the development of best-evidence guidelines, protocols and other governance measures, alongside increasing managerial control (Kuhlmann and Saks, 2008; Chamberlain, 2015, 2018). Equally, in the past, the neo-Weberian approach has demonstrated a tendency to berate the professions for their self-interested exercise of power, which has recently been reconsidered and found to be overly critical (Saks, 2016).

Saks's (2016) recent work provides a skilful and thoughtful analysis of the current relevance of neo–Weberian approaches, exploring a number of contemporary challenges to professional power in turn. As far as medicine is concerned, Saks notes a shift in power between medical specialists and generalists in the UK, with the latter attaining greater authority and influence at the policy level, as evidenced by the composition of clinical commissioning groups (CCGs), for example (Saks, 2016). This point has a bearing on the allied health professions considered here. In conclusion, Saks asserts that despite some criticisms, the neo–Weberian model continues to offer a robust theoretical framework for the analysis of professions and professional power. Therefore, it forms the key theoretical underpinning for this chapter.

Podiatry and foot surgery: from aspiration to regulation

The idea that podiatrists (then known as chiropodists) should be able to legitimately undertake invasive foot surgery would have been considered unthinkable 50 years ago (Larkin, 1983; Graham, 2006). Surgery was universally acknowledged as the exclusive domain of the medically qualified; practitioners became specialised in surgery by virtue of further extensive training and education, and were thus highly skilled. In contrast, Larkin (1983: 156) noted that state registration (in 1960) for UK chiropody acknowledged it as a legitimate, mainstream 'profession' but was based on both state support and medical approval, and the latter thus became a 'resource in the conflict–ridden low status world of footcare'. For Larkin (1983: 156), writing about allied health professions newly registered in 1960, the role boundaries of the allied health professions 'represent not what enhances their market power but what limits their challenge to medicine'. How, then, did the profession of chiropody so dramatically alter course and achieve regulatory approval for a specialism that so clearly encroached on a core part of medical practice? At what point did it even consider itself capable of an expansion in scope of practice that would enable surgical practice, and how did it achieve it?

By the late 1960s, the relative absence of innovations in practice had led to a degree of disenchantment among several practitioners, who looked at dentistry as a model to which to aspire (Borthwick, 2005; Graham, 2006). Dentistry was viewed as a successful profession, yet with a similar background to chiropody, reflecting a similar skill set, having a focus on a discrete part of the body and employing similar practices using forms of instrumentation familiar to chiropodists themselves (Graham, 2006). It differed in that it enjoyed not only full professional status recognised through an Act of Parliament, but also a university-degree education like medicine.

In an attempt to emulate dentistry, a small group of chiropodists based in Croydon, a suburban area of South-west London, decided to introduce a new modality to practice in the form of injectable local anaesthetics (Borthwick, 2005). At the time, this was a radical departure from the recognised scope of practice and was initially rejected by both the professional body and the regulatory body once news of its use had reached them (Borthwick, 2005). Intriguingly, most of those using the techniques had been 'trained' in them while serving in the medical corps of the British Army as part of National Service through the 1950s. Their role in the Army Medical Corps was that of medical orderlies, which therefore included tasks outside the scope of chiropodists in civilian life (Borthwick, 2005).

The fact that these podiatrists were free to adopt such techniques reflected the basis of English common law. Common law provided one key advantage over Roman law, which is applied throughout most of Europe, in that it adopted the principle of 'caveat emptor', whereby only specific legislation would debar the right to perform medical practices (Editorial, 2000). In short, chiropodists (or anyone else) could undertake any procedure or treatment unless the law specified otherwise. Intriguingly, in Roman law, any practice of a type likely to carry significant risks to its recipients is debarred, unless there is a law that specifically allows it (for example, such as 'controlled' or 'authorised acts' in Ontarian law [Regulation of Health Professions Act 1991]). One obvious advantage to UK professions wishing to expand their scope of practice is that they may do so providing that they are able to justify it in a court of law should they subsequently be involved in a case of malpractice litigation (Montgomery, 2000). In other words, the consequences of undertaking an act of practice without being demonstrably competent in it may still be very significant. For podiatrists, surgery was thus possible providing that they could demonstrate competence (and adequate training and education) should they be held to account for their actions in court.

However, for the chiropodists seeking to use local anaesthetic agents, there was a legal obstacle – the UK Medicines Act 1960. This Act of Parliament, instituted as a response to the thalidomide crisis, identified local anaesthetic drugs as 'prescription-only medicines', a type of licensed drug that was only available to doctors, dentists and vets (Borthwick, 2000, 2005). Thus, the introduction of injectable local anaesthesia into the scope of practice for chiropodists in the 1960s required changes to legislation, and not merely a need to persuade the regulatory and professional bodies to support it. To complete that trio of tasks successfully took time, with much persuasion and lobbying involved. Indeed, the first courses in local anaesthesia run by the local Croydon group started in 1969, with continuing use of the drugs possible until the law was fully clarified in 1980, when a statutory instrument was enacted to finally permit chiropodists access to some (but not all) of them (Borthwick, 2001a, 2001b). By then, the group had been practising invasive bone surgery since 1971 (Borthwick, 2001a, 2005; Graham, 2006). Initially, this was undertaken in the private sector, without the knowledge or approval of the formal medical authorities.

Again, the move from using local anaesthesia to practising actual bone surgery – legitimately, within mainstream healthcare provision – required the approval of the professional body and the regulatory authorities, and would be likely to provoke a response from the medical authorities. The exercise of medical power and dominance was, however, counterbalanced by a shift in health policy and a resurgent political neo-liberalism, which opposed monopolisation and favoured competition (Ham, 2004; Nancarrow and Borthwick, 2005). The scene was set for a contest between the power of the medical profession and the values of marketisation. But how did UK chiropodists acquire the skill and confidence to undertake invasive foot surgery when it did not form part of their own training and education as registrant podiatrists?

See one, do one: the origins of podiatric surgery in the UK

Within five years of running its first course in local anaesthetic techniques, the local self-styled Croydon 'postgraduate group' had become a national professional body, the Podiatry Association. It became the representative body for those practising podiatric surgery, as well as a provider of surgical training (Borthwick, 2000, 2001b, 2005; Graham, 2006). How did it achieve this transition so speedily? First, it imported surgical tutors from the US, where podiatric surgical practice already existed, albeit in a very limited form (Borthwick, 2001b; Graham, 2006). Its key resource, at least initially, was Jack Powers, a Californian podiatrist who was able to demonstrate two procedures: hammer toe corrections and nail removal with ablation using galvanic current (Borthwick, 2001b). Having witnessed the procedures being performed, the founders of the group then performed them, under Powers's supervision. This 'see one, do one' method of skill acquisition (as described by one of the founder members of the group) was the basis of the early emergence of podiatric surgery in the UK. It was carried out in the private sector, under the radar of the NHS medical authorities. Having acquired the skills, supplemented by occasional trips to the US for further informal training, the founding members became surgical tutors themselves, and established an education and training programme that was dependent on sympathetic and cooperative medical practitioners for its successful delivery. As interest in the group's activities grew, the founders decided to form a national professional body of its own, and chose to use the term 'podiatry' rather than chiropody in its title – the Podiatry Association (Borthwick, 2001b; Graham, 2006). Suitable medical allies were secured through the payment of fees offered for their services, and by the realisation that those seeking to develop such skills were both genuine and credible in their practices (Borthwick, 2001b; Graham, 2006). However, once the official medical authorities became aware of the existence of 'podiatrists', opposition grew (Borthwick, 2001b; Graham, 2006).

As the events unfolded, the key audiences in the drama emerged, most notably, the medical authorities (in the form of the British Orthopaedic Association, the Royal College of Surgeons of England and the Joint Consultants Committee of the BMA), the state registration board (the Chiropodists Board of the Council for the Professions Supplementary to Medicine [CPSM]) and the professional body (the Society of Chiropodists). Each had its own interests, and the dynamic between the three key factions ultimately set the scene for future practice.

Initially, the professional body (the Society of Chiropodists) sought to maintain cordial relations with the medical authorities, upon which it depended for support of its training and education in the 'schools of chiropody'. These were recognised for the purposes of state registration, and represented the legitimate face of chiropody, being sanctioned by the state and approved by the medical profession. However, it achieved this arrangement at the cost of subordination to the medical profession, which had essentially ensured a limited scope of practice (Larkin, 1983).

The regulatory body, the CPSM, had been established through legislation, and afforded legitimacy and orthodox recognition to the registrant professions (Larkin, 1983). As a regulator, it set standards and monitored practice, with the authority to approve scopes of practice. Each registrant profession at that time had its own board, which was populated by a mix of individuals from within the profession, as well as members from the medical profession. By 1979, the Chiropodists Board of the CPSM sought clarification from the Podiatry Association, whose members were all registrant chiropodists, on its surgical activities and its relations with medicine.

In 1980, the Royal College of Surgeons of England and the British Orthopaedic Association sought to limit chiropody to the scope of practice imposed on the profession in 1938, under the terms of the Board of Registration of Medical Auxiliaries, a voluntary register run by the BMA. Such a move was felt by the professional body (the Society of Chiropodists) to be virtually Dickensian, and it rejected the proposal; however, it also sought to compromise in order to safeguard medical support for existing training and education, and to maintain its standing as an established part of the health workforce (Borthwick, 2001b). The Royal College of Surgeons of England agreed to negotiate but, critically, the Chiropodists Board asserted its right to determine scope of practice as the legitimate statutory body with the necessary powers invested in it. With considerable insight, the Podiatry Association recognised the power of the regulatory body to outweigh that of the medical profession, and successfully ensured some of its own members were elected to the Chiropodists Board. With an influence inside the regulatory body, the Podiatry Association not only weathered the storm, but also ultimately ensured formal recognition by the state board via the addition of its own members to the register and recognition of 'ambulatory foot surgery' (Borthwick, 2001b).

From the margins to mainstream: establishing podiatric surgery in the National Health Service

Although achieving a foothold in practice through state recognition, convincing the medical profession to cooperate in establishing podiatric surgery as a viable service provision within the NHS was another matter. Yet, it proved possible because of a shift in health policy under a new government – one that favoured neo-liberal values and sought value for money in health service provision through the introduction of an 'internal market' (Malin et al, 2002).

Up until then, the health service had been run by consensus management, and the authority of the medical profession remained largely intact and unquestioned (Malin et al, 2002; Ham, 2004). Established hierarchies were respected and the professions were essentially monopoly suppliers. Margaret Thatcher's neo-liberal brand of conservatism instigated changes throughout the 1980s that altered the landscape entirely, emphasising general management reforms in the NHS (Cox, 1991). Not only did the subsequent government (under John Major) introduce a market structure for the health service, through a 'purchaser–provider' split (Cox, 1991), but it also invested in a system of general management, where key decisions would be made by executives empowered to manage it. In addition, general medical practitioners (GPs) were granted new powers to act as purchasers of services, through a system of fundholding; individual or groups of GPs would identify need and purchase services accordingly, while being encouraged to seek the best possible value for money.

Underlying such a structure and ethos was the principle of competition, where health service providers would compete to provide services. In order to be successful, they would need to demonstrate cost effectiveness, accessibility and clinical effectiveness. It was, therefore, a marketplace in which different providers of the same types of services would not only be allowed to exist, but also be encouraged to compete. General managers were empowered to decide on the selection of services, and GP fundholders were encouraged to think and behave as businesspeople. In such a climate, podiatric surgery was able to gain acceptance and legitimacy. Although formally opposed by the British Orthopaedic Association and the Royal College of Surgeons of England, podiatric surgery was an appealing option for many fundholding GPs on the grounds that it was effective, available, easily accessible (more so than orthopaedic surgery) and, as it operated on a day-surgery basis, often cheaper to provide. To illustrate the point, the Royal College of Surgeons of England commissioned one of its reports (Commission on the Provision of Surgical Services) on hospital-based foot surgery, which concluded that podiatric surgery was an effective and accessible option, and the Department of Health's own report ('Feet first', 1994) arrived at a similar judgement.

What followed was further action by the Royal College of Surgeons of England and the BMA's Joint Consultants Committee to limit the expansionist activities of podiatrists, only with one key difference. Having recognised that it was no longer viable to seek to prevent the development of podiatric surgery, it aimed thereafter to control it through incorporation and delegation (Borthwick, 2000). The focus of attention was shifted to suggest that podiatric surgeons, as 'non-medically qualified' practitioners, should ultimately work under the supervision of orthopaedic surgeons as part of an integrated team within the NHS. When this was resisted, the medical authorities questioned the use by podiatric surgeons of the title 'podiatric surgeon'. Certainly, the title 'surgeon' was protected under the Medical Act 1983 and was thus assumed to be exclusive to medically qualified surgeons. However, this was ambiguous, particularly as the use of a prefix – 'podiatric' – appeared to make it clear that the practitioner was a podiatrist trained in foot surgery, and not a medically qualified surgeon.

Coupled with the advent of managerialism and a marketised health service, the opportunity for podiatric surgery to become established and to thrive within the mainstream NHS grew. In reducing medical exclusivity and exposing the professions to competition, alternatives to existing service provision were embraced, providing they were financially competitive, easily accessible and safe.

However, this is not to suggest that medical power was so diminished that it was unable to influence policy; rather, it needed to regroup and recast its arguments in light of the policy agenda and prevalent political ideology. Today, calls for integrated and multidisciplinary care that are both flexible and responsive to need, require that podiatric surgeons also demonstrate a willingness to work with orthopaedic or other medical colleagues.

Most recently, attempts by the professional body in podiatry to have podiatric surgery regulated as a separate annotated specialism by the HCPC has brought these issues to the fore once more. Until January 2020, podiatric surgeons were simply registered as 'podiatrists' with the state regulator, along with those who did not practise foot surgery. It was not identified as a distinct speciality requiring further training and higher standards to ensure state recognition. By attempting to attain special annotation, the profession was seeking greater legitimacy for podiatric surgery, and thus to finally establish it as a recognised, regulated and independent provider of foot surgery. In finally achieving that status on 31 January 2020, it became a separately registered specialism, independently regulated and recognised by the state (see: www.hcpc-uk.org/media-centre/press-releases/2020/new-annotation-to-the-register-for-podiatrists/).

One element of the requirement to achieve annotation was to accredit the education and training programme with the regulatory body, the HCPC. In wishing to ensure independent expertise to assist in the accreditation process, the HCPC turned to the British Orthopaedic Foot Surgery Society, giving it a place on the accreditation panel. A considerable number of requirements and conditions were placed on the university seeking to accredit the programme, which may have reflected medical concerns over approving such independence in surgical practice by a non-medically qualified profession. Certainly, orthopaedic involvement in the accreditation panel suggests that the medical profession continues to exercise a degree of influence, giving substance to the theoretical importance of both cultural and social authority as a basis of medical power. Annotation also reveals the gender divide within the speciality of podiatric surgery in the UK; for a broader profession that has a marginally greater number of females than males, it is striking that its surgical speciality, based on figures from the College of Podiatry, is only 18 per cent female in composition.

Professional titles as 'symbolic capital'

Having largely exhausted all avenues in attempting to exclude, contain or control podiatric surgery, the medical profession sought to defend one last symbol of exclusivity and power – the use of title. While accepting, albeit reluctantly, the integration of podiatric surgery into mainstream NHS service provision, and acknowledging, however grudgingly, the technical competence of those practising podiatric surgery, there remained the issue of what they should be called (Laing et al, 2007).

The persistent use of the title 'podiatric surgeon', it was argued, would mislead patients, who would naturally assume podiatric surgeons to be medically qualified (Jerjes, 2011). Was it unreasonable to ask podiatrists practising surgery to use another title instead? At the heart of this conundrum lay the question of who had the right to refer to themselves as a surgeon (Menz et al, 2010). The Medical Act 1983 clearly restricted the title 'surgeon' to medically qualified practitioners. However, there were also examples where, if suitably prefixed, the term might be used to describe a different profession, for example, 'dental surgeon' was a title granted by the Dentists Act 1879 to dentists practising oral surgery, and few people today give much thought to the title 'tree surgeon'. The Medical Act 1983 includes a 'holding out' clause, which renders anyone in breach of the act if they 'falsely or wilfully' imply that they are medically qualified. Thus, the onus is on the practitioner to make it clear that in using a given title, they are not attempting to pass themselves off as medically qualified if they are not. If, then, a non-medically qualified professional was to prefix the term 'surgeon' with a term that gave a clear indication of their own professional background, would that suffice? Using this logic, the title 'podiatric surgeon' makes clear that the practitioner is a podiatrist who practices surgery, and not a medically qualified surgeon.

In the absence of a formal legal ruling on the matter, orthopaedic surgeons raised this issue publicly in the press to raise awareness of their concerns. In doing so, they attempted to devalue those using the title 'podiatric surgeon'. Bourdieu's notion of 'symbolic violence' provides a useful explanatory framework to understand the nature and importance of title in preserving power and social capital, and his grasp of the way in which titles are defended is mirrored in this exemplar.

Symbolic violence refers to the subtle way in which power is exerted without appearing to be so – it is achieved by an appeal to take the 'ordinary order' for granted, so that it seems obvious and unremarkable (Bourdieu, 1985; Bourdieu and Passeron, 1990; Menz et al, 2010). In this instance, it hinged on the likelihood of a public assumption that anyone who carries out surgery must obviously be medically qualified because it had always been thus; indeed, it would be unthinkable for it to be otherwise. Pejorative terms were assigned to those perceived to be breaching this obvious 'fact'; thus, podiatric surgeons were 'hijackers', as well as 'pseudoscientists' that would 'mislead', 'hoodwink' and 'deceive' patients (Borthwick et al, 2015: 316).

Such derision is characteristic of Bourdieu's concept of symbolic devaluation: the means by which a competitor (usurper) is 'objectively devalued' by the current, legitimated, holder of the prestigious title (Borthwick, 2015). Why such a fuss over mere title? As Bourdieu (1985: 733) explains: 'it is not the relative value of the work that determines the value of the name, but the institutionalised value of the title that can be used as a means of defending or maintaining the value of the work'. This has a powerful resonance in the modern world of healthcare professionalism given the loss of exclusivity of role and work tasks, and the policy desire for workforce flexibility and the blurring of boundaries that might threaten existing hierarchies of prestige.

Allied health professions as prescribers of medicines

Unlike the preceding example, the right to prescribe medicines has been restricted by statute in the UK since the enactment of the Medicines Act 1968. Thus, for allied health professions to become legitimate prescribers required a change in legislation, as well as an ability to convince others of their ability to do so safely and effectively.

In stark contrast to medicine and dentistry, the allied health professions were excluded from consideration when the current medicines legislation was first enacted in 1968. It was established, in part, as a response to a crisis resulting from the consequences of thalidomide use, in which the children of pregnant mothers taking the drug were born with teratogenic deformities (Borthwick, 2001a). By raising standards and tightening regulations, it sought to prevent any similar scandal in future. As a result, the strict regulatory framework of the Act not only established new categories of medicines (reflecting their relative risk), but also determined which professionals should have access to these medicines. Prescription-only medicines – one of the new categories introduced to signify medicines of higher risk – were strictly limited to doctors of medicine, dentists and vets. No other profession was considered likely to use these medicines as part of their everyday practice. It therefore followed that the allied health professions (and nursing) were automatically excluded from access to prescription-only medicines, as well as pharmacy-only medicines (a slightly less risky category). They were merely permitted to access those medicines deemed to be of such low risk that members of the general public were able to purchase them (general sales-list medicines). Allied health professions were thus assigned a level of competence equal to that of any member of the general public. Although registered as 'professionals' under the relatively new Professions Supplementary to Medicine Act 1960, most allied health professions were regarded as support staff for medicine, and not in any way adequately trained or educated to assume roles with such responsibility as the prescription or supply of medicines. It was clearly going to be an uphill struggle to change this mindset, and so it proved. Nor was this mindset unique to UK allied health – allied health profession prescribing in Australia largely mirrored the experience in the UK (Gilheany and Borthwick, 2009).

From zero to hero: the shift towards physiotherapy, podiatry and radiography prescribing

Between 1968 (when the Medicines Act received Royal Assent) and 1980, none of the allied health professions had secured any legislative change to enable access to the restricted categories of medicine, though not for want of trying. Podiatry, for example, fought a long campaign during those years to obtain rights to a handful of local anaesthetics agents. They had previously been able to access these medicines, but after the Medicines Act 1968 came into effect, the door was closed. Later, after the regulatory body had changed its view and agreed to recognise 'local anaesthetic techniques', it then took a further eight years to gain the support of the Department of Health and the Medicines Commission for an 'exemption list' of medicines. In full, there were only four prescription-only local anaesthetics on the list, in addition to a small list of pharmacy-only agents. Statutory instruments were used to grant access to these medicines, which thus constituted a formal 'exemption' from the terms of the Medicines Act 1968. 'Exemptions' became the first vehicle for allied health practitioners to obtain rights to administer and to supply restricted category medicines. Podiatrists were provided with the first exemption for 'administration' purposes in 1980 as local anaesthetics were injectable medicines, and thus administered by the practitioner rather than supplied by them to the patient. Only nurses and paramedics had acquired similar rights at that time, and it was only in 1998 that podiatrists were able to extend the list to include medicines for sale and supply (as opposed to administration) – though only to five in total. Thus, after a further period of 18 years of lobbying, podiatrists had only marginally extended access to prescription-only medicines. This was to change very rapidly.

By the late 1990s, it became apparent that the UK's demographic profile meant an ageing population with fewer younger people entering the workforce to compensate for the losses to retirement and age-related ill health (Cameron and Masterson, 2003). Policy shifted to address the problem, and an erosion of professional boundaries was ushered in by a Labour government intent on creating a flexible, adaptable workforce. Work roles and tasks that were previously exclusive were to be opened to other providers. In the wake of the marketisation of health services by the earlier Conservative governments, 'breaking down professional barriers' seemed a natural progression (Department of Health, 2000).

In 1999, June Crown published a report on the *Review of Prescribing, Supply and Administration of Medicines* (Department of Health, 1999), which acknowledged that new groups of professions would be considered as potentially able to prescribe in specific identified clinical areas. It specified two key categories of prescriber – 'independent' and 'dependent' – and named those professions it recommended as early candidates for progression to prescriber status. For the very first time, three key allied health professions were included as potential independent prescribers: optometrists, specialist physiotherapists and podiatrists. These recommendations were accepted by the government, and a series of staged extensions to prescriber status ensued. Pharmacists and nurses led the way given their high numbers, and were followed, as envisaged, by the allied health professions. In 2000, the additional mechanism of group protocols was given legal status as PGDs, allowing certain categories of prescription-only medicines to be supplied by allied health professions for specified categories of patients (such as people with 'diabetic foot infections'). However, it was in 2005 that the first prescribers emerged; initially, these were 'supplementary prescribers' ('dependent prescribers' in the Crown Report), who had to follow a regime initiated by a medical doctor but with authority to monitor and prescribe within a pre-existing and approved 'clinical management plan'. Physiotherapists, radiographers and podiatrists were the first allied health profession supplementary prescribers. 'Extended formulary' nurse practitioners and pharmacists were then granted independent prescriber status the following year (in 2006). By 2008, there were only 96 physiotherapy, 64 podiatry and 16 radiography supplementary prescribers on the register, but growth was steady. That same year, the Department of Health's Chief Allied Health Professions Officer initiated a scoping project, to conclude within a year, which would explore the need for a further extension in prescribing rights (Department of Health, 2009). Its most notable conclusion was that there were good grounds for seeking an extension to the level of independent prescribing for podiatrists and physiotherapists. In effect, this would be the test case to see if the allied health professions would be accepted as independently able to prescribe medicines. It was not to be an easy journey. The subsequent Department of Health Allied Health Professions Medicines Project took a further two years to make its final submission before the full CHM, with legislation coming into effect later in 2013.

In itself, the process played out in classic neo-Weberian fashion, with the key competing interests of state, medicine and allied health clashing. Unlike on previous occasions, the CHM required two subcommittee submissions to precede the full submission – one for podiatry and one for physiotherapy. Both proved difficult and challenging. Prior to the full submission, it was evident that acceptance was anything but a foregone conclusion. It was also clear that the CHM panel needed considerable reassurance that the allied health professions of physiotherapy and podiatry would be safe prescribing practitioners, and that they were sufficiently educated to be able to undertake prescribing training effectively and successfully. Considering that nurse and pharmacy prescribing had already been accepted and was in place, and that a common set of competencies was required of all prescribing professions (including medicine and dentistry), the reticence to agree to allied health independent prescribing seemed to betray a belief that allied health professions were less well qualified and prepared than either nurses or pharmacists. By 2015, this anxiety was further evidenced by the rejection of paramedic and radiography independent prescribing by the CHM. Any broader sense of a gradual 'natural' expansion of prescribing to a wider group of competent allied health professions as part of the solution to the growing workforce shortages was sharply disabused. Nor did independent prescribing for the nursing, pharmacy or allied health professions constitute an equivalent to medical doctor prescribing, despite the allusion to it in the title. Its terms lacked the full scope of doctor prescribing, omitting access to unlicensed medicines or the full range of controlled drugs (the equivalent of schedule 8 drugs in Australia). The latter was restricted to a list of four controlled drugs for podiatrists and seven for physiotherapists. As final arbiters of prescribing rights, the CHM demonstrated a clear anxiety and reluctance to recognise so many autonomous, small and niche professional groups as sufficiently competent and safe to grant full rights to prescribe independently. What is so striking is that this occurred at a time when the broader health policy agenda called for innovative solutions to the demographic challenges and workforce shortages that were clearly emerging and were evidently set to deepen over the decades ahead. However, resubmissions by these professions were partially successful (two years later), though they served as a sharp reminder of the need to demonstrate good governance, high levels of education and effective accountability.

Allied health prescribing: current issues

By 2017, the focus of attention moved to further changes in legislation to allow these groups (physiotherapy, podiatry and paramedics) further access to controlled drugs. One drawback of being restricted to a specific list, enshrined in statute, is that it will tend to date very quickly as assigning a drug to a given class of medicine does not necessarily mean that it will remain there in perpetuity. Some drugs and preparations are deregulated, and others moved to higher-risk categories, depending on political as well as clinical considerations. Political and public concerns about the overuse of opioid drugs may influence widening access to these drugs to a broader range of professionals. Recently, due to such concerns, certain drugs that allied health profession independent prescribers had been accustomed to prescribing were reclassified as 'controlled drugs'. As a result, they were no longer available to allied health profession independent prescribers. To render them accessible would require a change in legislation. However, broad concerns over the misuse of opioid drugs leading to addiction because of overprescription – the 'opioid epidemic' – may hamper support. In such a climate, it is reasonable to assume that the authorities might be disinclined to widen access to an even greater number of possible prescribers. It is equally possible that as more and more medicines are reclassified to the higher-risk 'controlled drug' category, allied health professions will experience reduced prescribing authority.

Allied health prescribing in Australia appears to mirror much of what is currently unfolding in the UK, with endorsement of prescribing registration following graduation within a year (approved from 1 August 2018) (see: www.podiatryboard.gov.au/Registration-Endorsement/Endorsement-Scheduled-Medicines.aspx). Similarly, in the UK, nurse regulators have considered moves to ensure new graduates are 'prescriber-ready' (all theory elements are to be taught at undergraduate level), with the practical 'prescribing in practice' being carried out within a year of graduation. In addition, pharmacy nurse and allied health programmes will no longer require a 'designated medical practitioner' to support the latter part as they now possess sufficient capacity to provide their own mentors. Parallel developments in the UK and Australia are most evident in this area, and probably reflect similar workforce pressures, demographic changes and recruitment issues.

One of the most revealing aspects of allied health prescribing is the way in which it is arranged, organised and funded in the UK. First, in order to apply to a programme, an individual practitioner is required to have the approval of an employer. This also involves having a prearranged and agreed medical mentor, who will undertake the role in the practical assessment module. Thus, an employer must first determine whether there is an identified need for a prescriber within the organisation. Usually set within an NHS trust, this means that there is direct managerial oversight of the entire process.

If the employer decides there is an identified need for a 'non-medical prescriber' in a given field, then a training place may be commissioned. Various non-medical professionals may apply for the training place. If the role is within a musculoskeletal setting, it is conceivable that an eligible physiotherapist, podiatrist or nurse may apply for the funding. Which one receives the funding will be decided upon by the managers in possession of the budget. All of this is predetermined by the requirements specified in the Outline Curricular Framework documents for prescribing professions. Only in the private sector is there a degree of autonomous decision-making possible. In that example, where a podiatrist works as a single practitioner running a small business, the applicant to the course is also the employer. As the employer, the podiatrist may approve their own application. However, they must also find a suitable and willing 'designated medical practitioner' to provide mentorship in practice, which is often more problematic than is the case for NHS workers.

In recent times, commissioning of healthcare providers (in the NHS) occurred within CCGs in England, with GPs playing a central role. It is therefore clear that GPs, acting as both medical practitioners and managers, have the ultimate authority to select services to provide healthcare for the geographical area within their remit. Within the hierarchy of structure, it is equally clear that there is no formally assigned voice for allied health. Decisions on individual applications for prescribing programmes are not, of course, made at board level, but delegated to the multi-professional teams working within the units involved; however, the local strategy and policy is determined by CCG boards.

These case exemplars provide some evidence of the forces impacting on the allied health professions, and give an indication of the continuing relevance of the concepts of medical dominance, managerialism and deprofessionalisation. Although subject to conflicting accounts, there is evidence to suggest that New Public Management has had, and continues to exert, significant influence over the professions (Dent and Whitehead, 2002; Numerato et al, 2012; Salvatore et al, 2018). However, some authors contend that assigning such importance to managerialism alone is too simplistic, stressing effective counter-strategies adopted by the professions, such as reorganisation, re-stratification and relocation (Noordegraaf, 2016). Carvalho (2014) has suggested that professions have largely been successful in withstanding managerial control, while others, such as Evetts (2011), see the impact of managerialism as profound. Much depends on context. The same can be said for the deprofessionalisation thesis. As Saks (2015, 2016) has demonstrated, deprofessionalisation and managerial authority in medicine has been more obvious in the US as a result of managed care but rather less obvious in the UK's NHS (aside from enhanced state regulation). He notes the influence of re-stratification in shifting power within UK medicine as GPs increasingly assume managerial roles at the expense of hospital specialists.

But how have these forces influenced the allied health professions, and what can the case exemplars here tell us about their impact? As is argued elsewhere in this book, the development of internal hierarchies in the allied health professions may have afforded them a degree of protection from the erosive forces of deprofessionalisation and managerialism. This is perhaps especially the case where internal stratification (specialisation) has become established and formally or officially recognised. The practice of invasive foot surgery by podiatrists has shifted from a risky, marginal activity in the private sector to a formally annotated state-regulated activity. While it was vulnerable to attack by orthopaedic competitors in its early days, it has become less so as a result of formal recognition by the state. Perhaps reluctantly, the medical profession has had to accept the reality of podiatric surgery, even though it continues to disapprove of its use of 'medical' titles such as 'consultant' and 'podiatric surgeon'. Podiatric surgery appears to have successfully resisted medical dominance inasmuch as it has become a mainstream healthcare service provision, supported by the state. It has survived attempts to eliminate it, and to render it subject to medical oversight. Public expressions of disapproval by medicine are now largely limited to professional title rather than competency to practise. It was also accepted by the state at a time when neo-liberal values dominated policies designed to enhance competition and end long-established monopolies.

By providing relatively cheap day-surgery delivery in a timely manner, with good safety and outcomes data, podiatric surgeons have been able to earn contracts at the expense of overworked orthopaedic services with long waiting lists. Intriguingly, this did not mean absorption within hospital orthopaedic units, but led to a significant degree of independence and autonomy. Yet, the managers that purchased the services were often medical professionals who had become empowered through fundholding and, later, CCGs. In line with Saks's (2018) findings, it is the GPs who increasingly hold sway, enjoying the freedom to employ flexible, accessible and cost-efficient services, without being constrained by professional self-interests. Recent annotation of the speciality of podiatric surgery by the HCPC appears to have provided the final seal of state approval, allowing, in principle, a legitimate and sustainable provision into the future.

However, the allied health professions have not entirely escaped managerial control or the effects of medical hegemony. In the case of allied health prescribing, it has already been noted that the education and training of allied health profession prescribers is determined by service managers through commissioning (Borthwick et al, 2017). Managers assign a training place to a given allied health profession where a need is identified. Funding of the service is also a matter of managerial control. Although qualified to prescribe, an allied health profession prescriber working in a trust may be constrained by local formularies and immediate budgetary concerns, and even be required to refer patients to their GP for prescribing on occasion so that the costs are transferred to the GP budget (Borthwick et al, 2017). Allied health profession prescribing is not equivalent to doctor prescribing, yet the governance requires a common set of competencies in practice for all prescribers, medical and non-medical alike. Nor is there clear evidence to suggest that the addition of prescribing to the scope of practice of allied health professions has significantly enhanced professional status. In Australia, podiatrist prescribing is not covered by the insurance scheme (the Pharmaceutical Benefits Scheme), as it is for dentists and doctors. In some regions, allied health prescribing is still to be fully implemented, in spite of national legislation enabling it (Borthwick et al, 2010; Borthwick et al, 2017). Nevertheless, allied health professions are clearly seen as part of the solution to the workforce crisis, offering flexible options to service delivery.

Broadly, it appears as if allied health specialist fields of practice are valued as flexible and adaptable, being able to act as alternative sources of provision where medical services are scarce. In contrast, generalist allied health practice is clearly vulnerable to competition, erosion and genericism, as evidenced in initiatives such as the Calderdale Framework (Nancarrow et al, 2012). While allied health specialists such as podiatric surgeons or physiotherapy prescribers remain accessible, cost effective, competent and safe, they are likely to retain currency in the shifting landscape of healthcare provision because they bridge established professional boundaries. Prized as exemplars of flexible working, they remain lauded by policymakers as long as they fill the workforce gaps. However, they also remain strongly linked to their professional identities and are not immune from boundary encroachment. If they also engage in jurisdictional disputes with potential competitors, they may yet face the same fate.

SEVEN

Post-professionalism and allied health

This chapter examines the way the allied health workforce is being redefined and reshaped in the 21st century to respond to an increasingly complex healthcare delivery context. Specifically, we explore the way that new types of roles and workers have been systematically engineered through a process of disaggregation of health profession work into discrete tasks that are then reconfigured into new roles (Pain et al, 2018). We use the term 'post-professional' to describe this workforce (Randall and Kindiak, 2008; King et al, 2019). These new roles are designed to meet the needs of specific populations and may or may not align with traditional profession-based profiles and values.

This chapter explores the emergence of a growing 'post-professional' workforce, which comprises qualified health practitioners from a range of clinical backgrounds (typically allied health and nursing) who adopt new skills, either formally or informally, to become part of a new workforce with common skills and a shared title while also maintaining their primary profession. In other words, a range of existing professions actively codify and commodify new and/or existing tasks that are then adopted by other professional groups to form a new professional identity. These workers could be described as 'interprofessional practitioners' (Shield et al, 2006), as opposed to an interdisciplinary team, in which multiple practitioners come together to achieve a common goal. In some cases, these new identities are formalised into new roles, such as the diabetes educator, rural generalist or generalist mental health practitioner. In other cases, the roles may be less formal, such as assessment and case management roles.

The post-professional workforce described here is also distinct from transdisciplinary practice (Thylefors et al, 2005). Transdisciplinary practice assumes a high degree of role interdependence and role overlap between practitioners, and may rely on the transfer of codified tasks between practitioners; however, the practitioner retains their primary professional identity. This differs from the post-professional workforce, in which the worker develops a new, recognised identity based on the transferred tasks, which may be reinforced through training and the adoption of a new, common title.

The post-professional workforce has existing core training in a specific profession/discipline, and therefore has a primary professional identity, including the adoption of a common philosophy and principles of practice. The addition of the new tasks or skills enables these professionals to expand into a new area of practice and a new professional identity.

Much of the sociology of the health professions has examined health professions in the hospital context and in comparison to the medical profession (Wilensky, 1964; Freidson, 1970; Larkin, 1983; Willis, 1983). However, the hospital context is increasingly being replaced with new places and systems of working that change the organisational contexts of health delivery. Community-based care, delivering healthcare in patient's own homes and in rural and remote contexts, and the ability to use technology to deliver services remotely all change the interaction and relationships between the patient and the healthcare provider, as well as between different healthcare providers. The complexity of care is further compounded by the multiple, complex morbidities experienced by the community, requiring the input of multiple practitioners from across diverse agencies. These changing contexts have an important influence on worker roles.

The purpose of this chapter is to understand the contexts and drivers behind some allied health professions actively re-engineering their roles to form new professions. It appears that the allied health professions are actively involved in activities that have been described by other commentators as 'deprofessionalising'. However, to examine the allied health professions through a purely professional lens belies the complexity of the professions involved and the contexts in which they work.

A relatively unusual feature of the allied health professions is the extent of negotiated interdisciplinary and transdisciplinary working. While not unique to allied health, the allied health professions have a strong culture of working in multidisciplinary teams and they have developed tools to actively negotiate transdisciplinary working (Porter, 2014; Pighills et al, 2015). These inter/transdisciplinary relationships are important, in part, because of the niche areas of practice of the allied health professions. No single profession has the repertoire to meet all the needs of patients with complex, chronic illnesses. Instead, a range of practitioners with complementary skills come together in various configurations of multi/interdisciplinary relationships to respond to those needs. These interdisciplinary relationships can be negotiated at a team or institutional level but are also formalised into recognised training structures and professional hierarchies to form new, interprofessional roles to meet the specific needs of the target population. There are several formal and informal examples of such new roles, particularly in the fields of diabetes education, mental health and in generic assessment and case management roles, such as with the NDIS in Australia and with intermediate and transitional care for older people in the UK.

To explore the impact and implications of managerialism on the workforce in the 21st century, this chapter will examine two case studies of 'post-professional' workforces: the rural generalist allied health practitioner in Australia; and the diabetes educator role. We consider whether these roles are a type of deprofessionalisation (Haug, 1975) or post-professionalism (Kritzer, 1999), or a new type of workforce.

The concept of the post-professional workforce was first posed by Kritzer (1999), who outlined three features that determined post-professionalism:

- the loss of exclusivity over a unique area of practice;
- the segmentation of abstract knowledge as a result of increased specialisation; and
- the growth of technologies to access information resources.

As a consequence of these actions, tasks and roles that were previously the unique domain of specific professions can be delivered by a range of different practitioners, either as a delegated component of an auxiliary professional role or by being reconfigured to form a new type of profession or specialist role.

Haug (1975) described the deprofessionalisation of occupations as the loss of their unique qualities, such as their monopoly over knowledge, public belief in their service methods, authority over the client and autonomy. Haug attributed these changes to increasing accountability of the professions to the public and managers, as well as the democratisation of knowledge, which has closed the 'information gap' between the knowledge of the public and professionals, further eroding the professional monopoly on knowledge.

The codification and commodification of tasks by health professions can be examined through the 'technicality to indeterminacy ratio' proposed by Jamous and Peloille (1970), described in more detail in the Introduction. As Traynor (2009) points out, indeterminacy allows professions to emphasise the social qualities and experiences of their members that qualify them to make such judgements. However, technical knowledge has the attributes of verifiability and reproducibility, which provide a basis for scientific credibility and are an important basis of the evidence-based practice movement. Thus, insufficient technicality risks the scientific credibility of a profession.

The emergence of evidence-based practice in the early 1990s led to a rapid growth of systems to support the scientific credibility of professions through a 'technicising tendency', such as the development of clinical practice guidelines and professional competency frameworks and standards (Timmermans and Berg, 2010).

Of importance to this chapter is Jamous and Peloille's (1970) proposal that less powerful subgroups within professions or groups on the periphery of established professions are more likely to promote reforms based on increasing technicality. The allied health professions fall within this remit and have embraced technicality to different extents. For example, occupational therapists promote indeterminacy through their philosophy of occupation as a principle underlying their work, which distinguishes them from the pure technical aspects of their role (Nancarrow and Mackey, 2005), whereas physiotherapists are criticised for their almost exclusive focus on the biomedical model and treating the body as a machine, underpinned by a strong scientific/technical paradigm (Nicholls, 2018).

The technicising tendency has been strongly embraced by health professions. For instance, the introduction of the Agenda for Change (Department of Health, 2001) and *The NHS Knowledge and Skills Framework* (Department of Health, 2004c) provide an explicit mechanism for the appraisal of knowledge and skills by employers. The adoption of competency-based training is now widespread in the allied health professions (Speech Pathology Australia, 2001; Snyder et al, 2017), which relies on developing clearly codified professional attributes that can be systematically assessed. This has been taken further. For instance, the Victorian Department of Health and Human Services introduced a Credentialling, Competency and Capability Framework for allied health professionals working in Victoria. The framework was developed to explicitly codify and commodify areas of allied health practice for transfer between professions and organisations in order to enable allied health practitioners to respond to complex care environments and 'achieve optimal patient-centred care'. It aims to promote consistency across the workforce by 'promoting the development and transferability of capabilities and skills for the allied health workforce across diverse settings and occupational groups' (State of Victoria Department of Health and Human Services, 2016: 6). The risk of the focus on codifiable competencies is that it has the potential to privilege technical competence over 'aesthetic skills' because they are more amenable to rationalisation (Copnell, 2010).

The following case studies provide a valuable contrast of the different ways and structures in which new roles are emerging. The first case study is the credentialed diabetes educator (CDE) role, which is a highly structured, regulated role, initially established by the nursing profession but that has more recently provided entry for allied health professions to access the same training and title. However, there is evidence that the allied health professions have adopted this role in a different way to nurses due to the size, history and hierarchy of the nursing profession in comparison to the allied health disciplines. The second case study of the rural allied health generalist role in Australia concerns a highly structured, engineered role redesign process that was developed through the systematic analysis of tasks, patient needs and risks using a structured framework, the development of competencies around those tasks and their reallocation to different practitioners.

Interprofessional role boundaries of diabetes educators

This case study is based on King's analysis of the negotiation of interprofessional role boundaries within the diabetes educator role in Australia using a neo-Weberian lens (King et al, 2019). The study involved a literature review, documentary analysis and interviews with key stakeholders (King, 2018).

Diabetes educators are qualified health professionals who have completed additional training to support the self-management of people with diabetes in order to reduce the risks associated with the secondary complications of the disease. The history of diabetes educators was first documented in the US in the early 20th century, when nurses started to develop formal training and support programmes to help manage the consequences of diabetes through dietary management. The diabetes educator role was consolidated following the introduction of commercial insulin in 1922, which created a need for education and support programmes to help people with diabetes in the management of their insulin (Allen, 2003). While these programmes included the input of a range of professions, including podiatrists, it was not until the 1980s that the CDE role was formally introduced in Australia and North America.

The Australian Diabetes Educators Association (ADEA) was first established by nurses in 1981 (King et al, 2017a) and subsequently introduced the trademark title 'credentialed diabetes educator' in 1986. CDE status is attainable by professionals who have achieved specific criteria set out by the ADEA, including completion of an accredited postgraduate certificate course, mentoring with a CDE and participation in workplace learning. Initially, only nurses were eligible to train as diabetes educators; however, the ADEA has gradually allowed entry to dietitians, medical officers, podiatrists, pharmacists, exercise physiologists, midwives and physiotherapists (Australian Diabetes Educators Association, 2015a; King et al, 2017a). A similar, multidisciplinary model of diabetes education is recognised in the US, Canada and Germany, though not in the UK (Valentine et al, 2003; Ross et al, 2016).

We define the diabetes educator as a 'post-professional' role because a range of qualified professions from different disciplinary backgrounds assume the new and common title of 'credentialed diabetes educator' based on the adoption of agreed, shared competencies that are developed and endorsed by an external accrediting body (Kritzer, 1999; Nancarrow and Borthwick, 2005; King et al, 2019). Each member of the new profession (in this case, diabetes educators) retains their original professional identity but can also identify as, and be employed solely on the basis of, their new professional identity as a diabetes educator. Complexities arise from this role as a result of the way that professions from different backgrounds have embraced their new identity within their original professional repertoire and also the way they negotiate interprofessional hierarchies within their new role.

The scope of diabetes educators' practice is determined by a range of factors, including legislation, individual experience and training, available supervision, and the clinical context, as well as the primary profession of the practitioner (Australian Diabetes Educators Association, 2015b). While each profession brings a different perspective to the role, there are no legislated or regulated distinctions in scopes of practice between diabetes educators from different professional backgrounds. Despite this, in practice, the roles of nurses and allied health diabetes educators have been implemented and recognised differently (King et al, 2019). These differences illuminate some important features about post-professional roles that encompass a heterogeneous group of constituent professions.

An important difference in the treatment of allied health versus nurse diabetes educators was the preferential employment of nurse diabetes educators over allied health diabetes educators. This difference was reinforced by employers, such as hospitals, which advertise specifically for 'nurse diabetes educators' rather than a 'diabetes educator', establishing diabetes educator roles as nursing roles, rather than interdisciplinary roles. In contrast, the allied health practitioners in diabetes educator roles had often developed the role themselves in contexts where they were already working. This is likely to stem from the historic development of the diabetes educator role from a nursing background. King found evidence that some existing diabetes educators perceived that a nursing qualification was a prerequisite to be a qualified CDE (King et al, 2019). Such misconceptions limit the scope of and access to non-nursing diabetes educators.

One of the important differences in the way the diabetes educator role is enacted stems from the fact that diabetes education is incorporated into nursing as a sub-speciality but not by allied health practitioners. This, in part, reflects the fact that the nursing profession formally recognises internal hierarchies, such as advanced practice roles and nurse practitioners (Gardner et al, 2016), but allied health professions do not. Diabetes educator roles are often advertised as clinical nurse specialist or clinical nurse consultant, that is, a higher grade (and salary) than a general nurse position (King, 2018). Nurses working in the state system in diabetes educator roles are remunerated more highly that general nurses. In other words, the hierarchies within the nursing profession provide an infrastructure to embrace and incorporate new skills and repertoires that also serve to increase the status and rewards of the profession. The same structures are largely unavailable to the allied health professions.

In most Australian states, government-employed nursing professionals are employed under a single employment award that covers only the nursing profession. In contrast, the allied health professions tend to be employed under a large, collective award that is distinct from nursing and medicine. Similarly, nurses and midwives have their own unions and regulatory board, which are large, powerful lobby groups. In contrast, allied health professions are regulated individually and may choose to be members of a collective union within their state.

Accordingly, nurse diabetes educators benefit from the enhanced status, employment opportunities and income associated with this area of clinical practice (Nancarrow and Borthwick, 2005), none of which are apparent for allied health professionals working in this area. While some allied health profession groups recognise areas of extended practice or special interest, only podiatric surgery has achieved separate regulatory status in Australia and the UK (Borthwick, 2000).

This suggests that the large size of nursing and the internal hierarchies that enable specialisation help drive the professional project of nursing, and can be seen to reinforce nursing as a 'pure profession' (Noordegraaf, 2007). In other words, nursing can expand its professional repertoire by taking on new activities that expand the profession's scope of practice. This affords the profession increased status, rewards and authority that are not available to the allied health professions, who lack the same internal hierarchical structures. However, the lack of a professional hierarchy for the allied health professionals effectively results in 'horizontal substitution', or a widening of their scope of practice, without a concomitant increase in status or rewards, which could be defined as a hybrid profession.

A further difference between the allied health and nurse CDEs is a perception of differences in scope of practice. Diabetes educators with a nursing background have been perceived, at least by allied health professionals and nurses, to have a wider scope of practice than those with an allied health background with respect to medication management (King et al, 2017a, 2019). There was a historic misconception that nurses had legislative access to medication management that was not available to the allied health professionals. This was explained by the perception of the nurses that their roles were more holistic and framed around a caring framework in comparison with the allied health professions, whose roles are seen to be focused around niche areas of practice. King found that although nurses perceived that legislation was the point of delineation between their scope of practice and that of allied health professionals working in the diabetes educator role, this was not supported in practice because there was no legislation differentiating between nurse and allied health access to medication management.

Securing legislative role boundary reinforcement (state regulation) is considered the most decisive strategy of professional closure and is therefore commonly at the core of professional projects (Saks, 2010, 2012, 2014). However, attempts to secure legislative support are often met with resistance (Borthwick et al, 2010) and may be abandoned in favour of employing 'charismatic authority' to establish a formalised sub-speciality, much like diabetes specialist podiatrists have done in the UK (Bacon and Borthwick, 2013). King found that by adopting an authoritative position and reinforcing the perception of the legislative nature of role boundaries, whether these are legitimate or not, is an effective strategy of professional closure (King et al, 2019).

Finally, King also found that perceived role boundaries in diabetes education emanated from discursive strategies implemented by nurses. References to nursing values (holism, commitment, exposure and experience) and their relevance to diabetes education served to consolidate perceptions of role boundaries (Allen, 2000; Timmons and Tanner, 2004; Bochatay, 2018). While these non-codifiable qualities are not exclusive to nurses, there is an implication that allied health diabetes educators may not adhere to these values and, in turn, may not fulfil the role as effectively (Timmons and Tanner, 2004).

This perspective is important from a technicality to indeterminacy perspective (Jamous and Peloille, 1970), where nurses perceive that they have a monopoly on caring, which could be seen as the indeterminacy, whereas the allied health professions have gained their credibility in this field through their acquisition of the technical skills required to be a diabetes educator. In this example, the indeterminacy of the nurse's role is implied but it creates a power differential between the groups.

This case study presents an example of a post-professional role in which nurses have created a set of competencies for diabetes education that can be adopted by an agreed set of professionals. However, the ability of the groups to benefit from their post-professional status depends on the size and internal hierarchies of their primary professions. While there were no regulated differences in the scope of practice between the different professions, the nurses were able to incorporate the role into their professional repertoire in a way that enhanced their status, employability and income. This was enabled by internal hierarchies in the nursing profession that support specialisation. In contrast, the allied health professions, which are already, in effect, specialised professions due to their niche areas of practice, were unable to benefit professionally in the same way as the nursing profession and would potentially result in a hybrid profession. In addition, nurses have managed to maintain some authority through their size and hierarchies, as well as through an implicit indeterminacy around their caring function.

Rural allied health generalist model

The rural allied health generalist model was developed in Australia to address the well-documented problem of workforce shortages in rural and remote areas. It is generally accepted that rural and remote health practitioners require a broader skill base than metropolitan workers due, in part, to the varied client load, the complex workplace settings and the inability to sustain multiple speciality practitioners across smaller population groups (Nielson, 2014; Quilty et al, 2014). Rather than employing more allied health professionals to increase the skill mix, the rural generalist training equips existing individual allied health practitioners with a repertoire of skills in the form of a negotiated horizontal substitution of tasks between allied health practitioners from different professional backgrounds.

The Greater Northern Australia Regional Training Network (GNARTN) Rural and Remote Generalist: Allied Health Project was funded by the Australian government to develop training models for practitioners working in rural and remote areas (Nielson, 2014). The project was also designed to develop systems to create skill-sharing models for health services to adopt that were supported by appropriate risk management and governance structures.

The rural generalist allied health worker illustrates a post-professional occupation because, in this example, six allied health professions explicitly and cooperatively codified and commodified aspects of their roles and reallocated those roles to other professions and auxiliaries using a structured management tool to form a new rural generalist role. This process reinforces the importance of the balance between technicality and indeterminacy (Jamous and Peloille, 1970), in which the formalisation of technical tasks was seen to expose professions to external evaluation and control (Traynor, 2009). However, as opposed to the neo-Weberian approach to professional closure, in which professions seek to obtain a monopoly over discrete components of their work, the rural generalist model explicitly unpacks the technical aspects of work, leaving only the non-technical aspects untouched.

Most existing studies of interprofessional role negotiation explore the role dynamics between practitioners working within existing co-located teams (King et al, 2015), where role negotiation is dependent on a range of local contextual factors, such as the individual practitioners, the clinical requirements and the setting in which the care is provided (Nancarrow, 2004). The rural generalist project is unusual because it took place not at the team level, but across multiple organisations and jurisdictions. The goal was to develop a generalisable set of core, generic activities that could be reallocated across multiple professions, teams and services across a wide geographic area. This model has since been expanded and implemented by the Queensland government and formalised into a university training programme.

The context for the project was highly complex. Five teams across three states in rural and remote regions of Northern Australia participated in the project. The teams represented populations with diverse needs, such as Aboriginal populations, people with disabilities, ageing populations and people with rehabilitation needs. The services ranged from hospitals to remote outreach teams and included disability and rehabilitation services. Multiple agencies were involved, including Aboriginal Health Services, Medicare Locals (regionally based primary care organisations), hospitals and community-based health services. The allied health disciplines involved were occupational therapy, physiotherapy, speech language pathology, dietetics and nutrition, podiatry, social work, and allied health assistants.

The project involved staff from all professions across all of the participating services, who undertook a process of task codification and disaggregation using a structured workforce planning tool called the Calderdale Framework (Smith and Duffy, 2010). The Calderdale Framework is a tool developed by allied health professionals in the NHS that provides a structured way for professions to allocate tasks based on the needs of patients, rather than on historic professional repertoires (Smith and Duffy, 2010; Pain et al, 2018). It involves a facilitated process that identifies and codifies tasks or competencies through working with clinicians to break down clinical interventions into defined functions and tasks, which are aggregated into categories such as 'fatigue and sleep', 'chronic disease management and prevention', 'neurological' and 'maternal health'.

The tasks were analysed according to the level of risk and skill associated with performing each task, and the frequency with which the task is performed. Using a consensus approach, practitioners then determined which tasks were appropriate to delegate to another worker, either through a delegation framework to auxiliary staff (such as allied health assistants or other support workers) or for skill sharing across different professions in a team. Those tasks deemed to be appropriate for delegation were then codified through the development of competencies relating to that task.

The project specified that only data pertaining to clinical tasks were analysed. Interestingly, non-clinical tasks (such as care coordination, administrative/operational tasks and student supervision) were excluded from the task reallocation process because non-clinical tasks were deemed essential to all professions, and therefore not considered to be negotiable across professional boundaries. These tasks align with the managerial roles considered by Noordegraaf (2007) and suggest that allied health professionals moving outside the traditional professional hierarchies of, say, hospital structures are bound by a common set of managerial tasks.

This explicit separation of clinical tasks from non-clinical skills further reinforces the technicality to indeterminacy model (Jamous and Peloille, 1970). In this case, the technical skills were explicitly codified for reallocation across professional boundaries, while the non-clinical skills were not disaggregated, but recognised as a core offering of the primary profession.

The participating allied health professions identified 337 unique tasks, of which 127 were deemed appropriate for skill sharing across allied health professional boundaries with appropriate training and governance support. A high proportion of tasks were identified as interdisciplinary tasks. Of those tasks that were identified as appropriate for skill sharing, 40 per cent were currently only performed by a single discipline, though 60 per cent were already performed by more than one discipline. Similarly, only a small proportion of tasks were perceived to be discipline-specific. For example, one fifth of occupational therapy tasks and a quarter of physiotherapy tasks were deemed to be unique to those disciplines. The project also identified many tasks performed by allied health professionals that could be delegated to the allied health assistant workforce, though few of the potentially delegable tasks were being delegated.

The discrete tasks were then reorganised not according to profession, but into functional or diagnostic categories that reflected the perceived needs of the client groups. These clusters included categories such as: activities of daily living (ADL) and function; mobility and transfers; prevention of foot morbidity in high-risk groups; children's development; cognition and perception; communication; psychosocial; fatigue, sleep and energy conservation; pressure care, skin and wounds; diet and nutrition; neuro-musculoskeletal and pain; cardiovascular fitness and exercise tolerance; and continence assessment and basic intervention. Following validation of these groupings by other allied health professionals, these clusters were designed to form the basis of future clinical training programmes for rural and remote allied health practitioners. The aggregated task clusters were then analysed to determine which of the six practitioners could contribute to the delivery of these activities. In more than half of the clusters, two or more professionals were considered to currently deliver those roles. For example, the ADL cluster incorporated the activities of: ADL screening and assessment; assessment of and prescribing home modifications; equipment relating to ADL and function; and functional training for ADL. All disciplines other than podiatry were considered to contribute to this cluster.

Rather than being threatened by potential loss of role boundaries, professional status and monopoly over specific tasks, the participating staff supported the project and processes of role negotiation between practitioners. Additionally, the project had interdisciplinary oversight through the project governance team. Most participants supported the notion of greater delegation by practitioners within the team. Feedback from participants suggested that far from being threatening, the process enabled staff to gain a greater understanding of each other's roles.

Under the guise of person-centred care, this case study challenges several of the accepted assumptions about professionalism. Where traditional literature on the sociology of the professions focuses on the exclusionary practices of professions (Abbott, 1988), this study used a structured, democratic, negotiated approach to identify a suite of tasks that could be shared by more than one profession, with strong support for this process by the six disciplines involved. Further, the tasks were regrouped around a series of clinical functions, rather than historic professional repertoires.

The explicit identification of a set of tasks, the attribution of a level of skill and risk to these tasks, and the renegotiation of these tasks challenges the very assumptions underpinning professionalism. Professional work is distinguished from non-professional work through the interweaving of occupational content and institutional control to establish occupational closure (Noordegraaf, 2007). In this case study, in the context of the rural shortages and under the guise of person-centred care, the professions codified their practice into tasks, which they then willingly redistributed based on skill and risk levels with the active support of the institution. The focus on patient-centred care in the rural context became the overriding priority of this group. In other words, the functional purpose of the team superseded the professional boundaries of the individual professions involved, a process described elsewhere as 'incorporation' (Carmel, 2006).

Several contextual factors enabled this model. At a macro, or systems, level, the regulatory system was an enabler of the task reallocation because none of the specific tasks identified was subject to regulation. As a result, there were no regulatory/legislative barriers to the task transfer. Further, this process has now been formalised into the Rural Allied Health Generalist Programme, which can lead to a postgraduate qualification. In this programme, the competencies have been codified and endorsed by each profession into modules that can be adopted by other professional groups as a postgraduate study.

At a meso level, the remote geography, coupled with dispersed, small populations, meant that a multidisciplinary team could not be sustained due to insufficient numbers of patients to provide a full workload for multiple different types of practitioners. Instead, the remote context created the need to introduce practitioners trained with a suite of skills to meet the specific needs of the target population, rather than armed only with the niche skills of their primary professional repertoire, or 'interdisciplinary practitioners'.

As this study illustrates, complex contexts, such as rural and regional health, or even home or community-based care services, particularly for older people with chronic illnesses and or people with some types of disabilities, tend to demand a broad skill set that can generally not be met by a single practitioner (Nancarrow, 2004). While these patients need multiple services, it is not always feasible or practical to send a multidisciplinary team into a persons' home; instead, individual practitioners who have adopted an interdisciplinary skill set have been developed. Complex chronic conditions that require the input of multidisciplinary teams also facilitate the need for a more generalist workforce. For example, generic mental health workers can include nurses, psychologists, social workers and occupational therapists.

The shift from pure professional to hybrid roles is enhanced by the changing geographies of healthcare (Milligan and Power, 2010), with an increasing trend to deliver care away from formal hospital settings and closer to the patient/service user in their own environment (Andrews and Evans, 2008). A great deal has been written about the importance and role of the hospital as an organising structure (Finn, 2008), as well as the way that professions both maintain their status and reinforce structural inequalities in the hospital setting. However, a large proportion of allied health care is provided in a range of diverse, non-hospital settings, including the community, correctional facilities, schools, patients' homes, non-health organisations, residential care facilities and sporting facilities, to mention only a few. In addition, allied health services may be funded by a wide range of agencies, including health, social care, not-for-profit agencies, education, corrective services and private industry, as well as individual, fee-for-service private practices.

The technical deconstruction of the roles was brokered by the application of specific managerial tools designed to reconstruct roles around patient risk and need (the Calderdale Framework). The unions and professional bodies did not oppose the localised experiment, thereby enabling the changes. In addition, the complex organisational contexts for the project meant that multiple agencies and settings needed to be considered in the task reallocation.

At a micro (individual profession and organisation) level, the rural generalist practitioner model was facilitated by a lack of professional hierarchies and a broadly homogeneous professional culture (all of the professions involved adhere to the biomedical model). These features are likely to have enhanced the willingness of the professionals to participate and consensually reallocate their roles to others. The availability of the supportive, cross-organisational infrastructure, including project management, institutional sponsorship and external funding, were essential in driving this project.

In this case study, the allied health professions are relatively equal in status, and the reallocation of tasks from one professional group to another does not bestow any increase or decrease in status to donor or recipient professions. The professions involved are state-funded (by a range of agencies), so there is no fee-for-service negotiation involved (that is, there is less competition). Interestingly, there are no regulatory boundaries around the reallocated tasks. This reinforces the notion that the 'core' roles, especially those occupied by more powerful professions (vertical substitution), are more likely to be contested and defended (Zetka, 2011) but the lower-status, more 'peripheral' tasks are more likely to be shared or shed (Hugman, 1991).

Discussion

Within the neo-Weberian tradition, professions are assumed to be dynamic, competitive and concerned with achieving professional closure by securing a monopoly around a niche area of practice. This enables professions to secure their social standing and recognition, access to employment, income, and authority (Saks, 2012). In contrast, the case studies presented in this chapter suggest a shifting paradigm among the allied health professions. Instead of combative protectionism, the professions have willingly codified their professional practice into competencies that are consensually reallocated to other professions. In many cases, these approaches have been supported, or indeed brokered, by the state. We suggest a number of reasons for this.

The first is that the allied health professions are vulnerable to encroachment because of their niche areas of practice, small size and lack of internal hierarchies. The allied health professions have evolved individually with a niche skill base to address specific issues. However, the managerial agenda, alongside the patient-centred care agenda, means that increasingly complex patient needs require practitioners with skills that may be beyond their professional repertoire. The need for an interdisciplinary role is enhanced by specific contexts, such as community-based settings of care, workforce shortages or the need to deliver wider services to smaller and/or more dispersed populations (Nancarrow, 2004). However, with a much larger profession and access to hierarchies, nurses have begun to adopt components of allied health work and incorporate them into their roles as a specialisation (for example, rehabilitation nurses) (Long et al, 2002). The lack of hierarchical specialisations in allied health means that the converse does not occur. Thus, we suggest that internal professional hierarchies and greater professional size have the effect of protecting the 'pure professional' status of occupation groups, whereas the specialised niches, relatively small sizes and lack of protected tasks of the allied health professions mean that their 'indeterminacy' is more likely to reflect the managerial goals of the context in which they are working than a unique professional value or skill set.

Low-risk, low-status and unregulated tasks lend themselves more strongly to task reallocation. The social bargain into which allied health entered with the medical profession meant that the tasks undertaken by allied health disciplines tend to be of little interest to the medical workforce, and are seen as being of little risk of encroachment on medical roles (Larkin, 1983). Few specific allied health tasks are regulated, and as the rural generalist project shows, a high proportion of tasks are already undertaken by several different allied health disciplines, which means that the allied health claims to professional monopoly are relatively weak. Areas of higher risk, or those involving specialised and expensive technology, skills or training, are less likely to be able to be substituted and more likely to be contested (Nancarrow and Borthwick, 2005). Similarly, the 'indeterminate' roles have a lower likelihood of substitution, as illustrated by the rural generalist study, in which only the technical tasks were explicitly substituted between professional groups. Allied health professions have strongly embraced the technicality of their professional repertoires in the form of competencies, which actively codifies practice into commodities that can be traded, delegated and absorbed by other professional groups in the absence of the value base of the profession. In contrast, the nursing profession has managed to maintain some of its indeterminacy through a discourse of holistic caring (King, 2018).

By definition, specialisation normally involves a division of labour, enabling workers to delegate components of their work to others in order to enable them to focus on the 'virtuoso' roles (Hugman, 1991). Features that enable a workforce to maintain a more specialised skill set include the provision of services with a high throughput, or a high volume of work in a specific area, enabling clinicians to focus their activities on a narrower range of interventions while remaining fully employed (Nancarrow, 2004). Interventions that involve greater acuity or risk, including the need for high-tech or high-cost equipment, tend to require staff who can bring a dedicated skill set focused on treating a condition with little margin for error (Courtenay et al, 2013).

Previous research in community rehabilitation settings identified several factors that facilitate more role sharing, or a more generalist workforce (Nancarrow, 2004). Lack of access to other practitioners caused by a more isolated setting of care, such as the patient's own home or rural/remote settings, can result in task sharing though necessity, whereas the availability of a wider diversity of practitioners will create more opportunities and impetus for task specialisation. Practitioners who undertake joint home visits are more likely to adopt collaborative task-sharing practices. A longer duration of care provides greater opportunity for more delegation of tasks to support workers, as well as more transfer of roles between therapists, whereas highly acute and shorter-term care for rapidly changing patient needs requires more regular input from specialised staff. Greater complexity but lower-risk and lower-acute interventions lend themselves better to devolution and substitution.

For patients with multiple, complex needs, there are several considerations around having multiple practitioners delivering care, as opposed to a single, skilled, interprofessional practitioner (Duckett, 2005). The costs of multiple practitioners and the logistics of coordinating care, as well as the availability of the individual areas of expertise, all need to be considered. While post-professionalism creates opportunities to develop a more flexible workforce to meet the needs of the patient, it raises questions about the nature of professionalisation and the importance of this to the patient.

Conclusion

In this book, we have illustrated that the allied health professions are innovative, responsive, nimble and able to adapt to a wide variety of changing population needs and organisational contexts. On the one hand, as illustrated by the example of the podiatric surgeons in Chapter 6, allied health professions have successfully used managerialism to contest one of the most highly protected domains of medicine – orthopaedic surgery. On the other, as the example of the OTA role suggests, managerialism is eroding the core philosophies of the allied health professions and replacing them with an emphasis on technically focused tasks and competencies. Further, where the dominant, neo-Weberian theories of the professions focus on the protection of a monopoly of knowledge, the allied health professions are actively and consensually involved in the disaggregation and codification of their work so that it can be transferred to other allied health professions and the support workforce.

Allied health professionals have also demonstrated that they can adapt to a range of different organisational and clinical contexts, adjusting their roles and responses accordingly. However, unlike their medical and nursing counterparts, which have large institutionalised hierarchies to support their roles, allied health professions are often moving outside their narrow clinical boundaries and across organisational and institutional settings without a clear structure to fortify them. Perhaps this reflects the shift from a pure profession towards a hybrid profession (Noordegraaf, 2007), which has flexible boundaries, adapts to a range of organisational contexts and responds to the needs of the clients with which they work. The implications of this shift for the allied health professions themselves are still unclear.

The value and meaning of the allied health collective

Despite the prolific use of the term 'allied health', our analysis brings us no closer to a unifying definition of the confederation of allied health professions. It is clear that allied health professionals are distinct from medicine and nursing; however, those professional boundaries are beginning to blur as allied health professions take on traditional medical roles, such as prescribing and point-of-care testing (Buss et al, 2019).

That the allied health professions have evolved into distinct professions is probably an artefact of timing and context. Larkin (1983) suggests that a different timing for professionalisation may have seen some allied health professions fall under the division of labour of nursing. Equally, it is possible that some roles, particularly optometry and possibly radiography, may have fallen under the medical division of labour rather than become autonomous allied health professionals in the absence of well-established professional associations.

There are several pragmatic reasons why the professional skill repertoires of each of the allied health professions have evolved as they have (Larkin, 1983). However, the active re-engineering of the workforce that is now taking place shows that many of the traditional professional models are not fit for purpose. The pursuit of the professional project and the early division of labour of the health professions have reinforced the individuality of the professions, and these have been supported and reinforced by state and self-regulatory structures. Yet, simultaneously, the allied health professions are actively rearranging their roles to fit new contexts and population needs.

The COVID-19 pandemic resulted in the rapid removal of legislative restrictions on some areas of scope of practice to allow allied health professionals to deliver tasks normally delivered by others in critical shortage areas (Bourgeault et al, 2020). Examples include: the training of allied health professionals to work in critical care in response to nursing shortages; reducing prescribing limitations for allied health practitioners with prescribing licences; and having podiatric surgeons manage orthopaedic medical wards to free up medical doctors. COVID-19 created an environment for legislative change that meant it was possible to rapidly and safely mobilise the whole health workforce during a time of crisis rather than the protection of professional titles and repertoires.

Before the COVID-19 crisis, similar questions about workforce flexibilities were being asked. For instance, Duckett (2005) pointed out that as people age and their needs become more complex, they need access to a wide range of different interventions, most of which cannot be delivered by a single practitioner. There are high costs associated with employing and coordinating multiple practitioners. Alternatively, we take other complex tools that disaggregate tasks from professions and reconfigure them into new 'interdisciplinary' roles. The 'allied health' collective is largely a way for bureaucracies to manage the complexity of the confederation of different workforces and has no clinical meaning.

The allied health umbrella provides opportunities to create a new and responsive workforce, as demonstrated by the emerging professions.

The allied health identity, supported by a self-regulation pathway, facilitates the professionalisation of new health workers who meet specific needs of the population. The example of the DEs was one of the few examples of where the pursuit of 'allied health' per se created a specific advantage for an occupational group.

What we can say conclusively about allied health is:

- They adhere to the medical model/orthodoxy, as distinct from complementary medicine, though some professions may operate within more of a social framework.
- Allied health professions perform a niche area of practice that meets a particular need in society (based on a certain body part, treatment modality, philosophy or population group).
- To become an allied health profession, occupations must have met a socially agreed standard for entry to a profession. These standards are not uniformly defined; however, in the UK, recognition as an 'allied health profession' is determined by regulation by the HCPC. In Australia, there is no uniform definition and the entry criteria are determined at a jurisdictional level; however, there is increasing consensus around entry standards, as defined by the AHPRA and the National Alliance of Self Regulating Health Professions (NSRHP).
- Allied health professions have evolved from a post-industrial and largely British colonial organisational framework that has shaped their interprofessional relationships, scopes of practice and workforce diversity.
- Diversity is a poorly developed area within the allied health literature. Ethnic diversity in the allied health professions tends to focus on strategies to reduce health inequalities, such as cultural competence, cultural safety and health literacy. Educational strategies predominantly focus on approaches to increasing the representation of minority ethnic groups in allied health training, or assimilation. An exception to this is the development of Aboriginal and Torres Strait Islander health practitioners, who constitute a registered professional group introduced to provide culturally safe clinical care services to Aboriginal and Torres Strait Islander people and communities by working alongside and collaboratively with other clinicians, including doctors, nurses, midwives, allied health and oral health practitioners in a range of settings.
- Allied health may have a broad individual clinical scope of practice or work in a more specialised role, depending on a range of factors, including the individual's qualifications and competence, practice

location, practice setting, level of supervision, and community need. They can assess, diagnose, treat, educate and use scheduled medicines depending on their approved individual scope of practice outlined in a practice plan.

- The allied health professions are a highly feminised workforce. Overall, the sociological literature suggests that the division of labour and employment settings are differentiated by gender and status, with males expressing a preference for more scientific, technical and sports-related tasks, more likely to work in more autonomous roles such as private practice, and pursuing management roles within bureaucracies. As with nursing, allied health professions are more likely to adopt more caring roles and work with more emotionally complex populations. There are profession-based and international variations that influence the gender and professional diversity and status of each allied health profession.

Allied health leadership and driving changes

Despite their largely successful professionalisation strategies, the allied health professions still face many challenges in influencing service delivery in a way that optimises the use of their services. An important finding from the Victorian Allied Health Workforce Research Project was that while there was unmet community need for allied health service provision, there was generally not a shortage of allied health workers in Victoria (and in some cases underemployment of allied health workers); rather, there was insufficient funding for service provision (see: www2.health.vic.gov.au/health-workforce/ allied-health-workforce/allied-health-research). This was believed to result from the perception that allied health is often a 'Cinderella service', suffering from chronic underfunding and the first to be cut when funding shortages arise. In the private sector, many professions reported market failure in the delivery of allied health services. In other words, it was difficult for allied health professionals to create a sustainable private practice business model to meet the needs of some communities, particularly regional, rural and low socio-economic status communities.

There is a substantial body of clinical evidence to support the effectiveness of many individual allied health interventions, for example, preventing readmission to hospital (Rogers et al, 2017), lowering the risk of falls (Spink et al, 2011), reducing the risk of discharge to residential aged care (Adams and Tochhini, 2015) and improving post-operative clinical outcomes (Boden et al, 2018), to mention only a few. However, research evidence tends to be fragmented by clinical field and by professional grouping, making it difficult to argue for the introduction of allied health interventions at a system level.

Several of those challenges stem from the confederated nature of the allied health professions and the heterogeneity of the practitioners brought together for pragmatic management reasons. This creates challenges of professional identity (individually and collectively), management, funding and organisation, which are reflected in the performance of allied health (Boyce and Jackway, 2016; Dawber et al, 2017; Bradd et al, 2018).

The relatively small size of individual allied health professions in comparison with, say, medicine and nursing limits their ability to advocate for their services and clients. For example, medicine and nursing have employment structures that enhance their ability to advocate and also create differential access to education and training in the employment setting (Boyce and Jackway, 2016; Nancarrow et al, 2017; Bradd et al, 2018). The employment of doctors and nurses is often the subject of high-profile political strategies (Han, 2018), but it is rare for allied health professions to form the basis of political lobbying.

A survey of senior leadership positions in Australian health organisations found that allied health professions are significantly under-represented in senior and executive management teams and health board positions where they have the opportunity to influence system performance, quality and safety (Boyce and Jackway, 2016). Boyce found that allied health professionals held only 3.4 per cent of Australian senior leadership positions, compared with 10.4 per cent for medicine and 9.3 per cent for nursing/midwifery. Of all national health board members with known qualifications, 6.3 per cent were allied health professionals, compared with 15.4 per cent for medicine and 8.1 per cent for nursing/midwifery.

Lack of exposure to management team positions, in turn, limits the capacity and capability of allied health professions to move into senior and executive leadership roles. Involvement of allied health in senior leadership positions provides the opportunity to contribute to policy decisions, as well as opportunities to work towards integrating allied health services into core health models (Mason, 2013).

Allied health professionals are largely trained and socialised to be members of a single profession, not an 'allied health professional'. However, almost uniquely for allied health professionals, as clinicians progress into leadership roles in larger organisations, their responsibilities shift from being a unidisciplinary practitioner to having to lead interdisciplinary teams and advocate for multiple professions (Boyce and

Jackway, 2016; Bradd et al, 2018; Smith et al, 2019). Boyce suggests that one solution is to leverage the roles of specific allied health leaders, for example, chief allied health officers, professors of allied health and directors of allied health, as agents of change deployed to create, shape and capture the allied health brand, and to lead the discursive strategies necessary to cement the allied health presence and demonstrate value to the state and other actors (Boyce and Jackway, 2016).

What the international comparisons teach us

The comparison of the professionalisation pathways of the allied health professions across two jurisdictions teaches us many things and is effectively a comparative case study. Despite many common origins to both the Australian and UK health systems, the divergence of the two systems after the Second World War created some significantly different contexts for the evolution of allied health.

The formation of the NHS in 1948 effectively created a large monopoly employer in healthcare. The regulation systems established in the mid-20th century and the Professions Supplementary to Medicine Act 1960 created a stable core of allied health professions that has largely remained to the present date. The centralised funding of roles and a single pay scale enabled the re-engineering of roles and tasks vertically and horizontally along a skills ladder. While this has not been fully realised, it has been centrally driven and created – largely uncontested – opportunities for workforce change. Examples include the roll-out of Agenda for Change in the early 2000s and the introduction of large-scale workforce programmes, such as the CWP (see Chapter 5), which saw the rapid prototyping and implementation of new roles such as support workers. In addition, the NHS was able to centrally drive the provision of innovations such as supplementary prescribing, largely overcoming the interprofessional tensions seen in Australia.

The other opportunity for the allied health professions under the NHS is that their professional organisation and their employer are closely aligned. This should give them opportunities to drive high-level changes because of their critical mass and large voice. In fact, there is little evidence of this.

A further defining feature of the UK NHS is the provision of almost all personal care through the health and social care portfolios. These portfolios help to create a singular definition of 'health' and 'social care', and, with few exceptions, most allied health is provided within the 'health' portfolio. The alignment of the regulation structures for allied health (the HCPC) with the NHS further reinforces the 'health' model of allied health. In comparison, healthcare provision is far less organised in Australia.

The Australian system, in contrast, is highly pluralistic and there is no legislatively endorsed central recognition of or endorsement for the collective allied health professions. The professions must operate within a more competitive funding environment, often competing directly against each other for patients. However, the corollary to this is that the mechanisms for allied health endorsement are far more flexible. New professions can emerge and persist relatively uncontested to meet population needs. Those that demonstrably adhere to a set of self-regulation guidelines can work with large state and private funding bodies to achieve co-regulation, and effectively social closure, giving them access to funding, as illustrated in Chapter 4.

It is unclear how, or whether, those same 'emerging' healthcare needs are met within the NHS system. Examples of relatively well-established professions elsewhere, such as exercise physiologists and diabetes educators, have had little traction within the UK market. Does this mean that those services are not being provided, or that they are being provided by others in different ways?

The health financing models in Australia, which largely provide funding to individual services/providers or service users, rather than block grants as in the NHS, create opportunities for innovation and entrepreneurship in healthcare. However, there are also risks of a 'race to the bottom' in terms of pricing and skills dilution through substitution to lower-cost, lower-skilled workers. This risk is particularly increased through the codification and delegation of tasks to new workers outside of the organising framework of a profession.

A common feature in both environments is that we have seen the relationship between medicine and the allied health professions evolve over the past century. As the defining relationship with the medical profession declines in importance, the relationship of the professions with the state increases in importance. In Australia, the relationship between the professions and the state has provided opportunities for professions to evolve. In the UK, it has provided opportunities for professions to interact/have internal flexibilities. However, the extent of medical interference in the growth of the allied health professions has been greater, and lasted longer, in Australia, with some influence still apparent. For example, non-medical prescribing was centrally coordinated when introduced in the UK, whereas state variations in legislation and different professional cultures led to inconsistencies in the uptake and extent of medical influence of prescribing in Australia. It makes sense that a more devolved market creates more interprofessional competition, particularly in the fee-for-service arena, as multiple practitioners compete for the same patient dollars.

Allied health and technology

Technology has been an important driver of innovation and change in the allied health professions. The professions of sonography, radiography, optometry, pedorthics, prosthetics and orthotics have either been heavily shaped by, or only exist because of, technological innovation over the past century. As technology becomes ubiquitous within everyday life, the technological drivers for change are increasingly rapidly.

There are multiple implications for allied health professions arising from the growth of technology. These include the opportunities to provide remote care. In other words, technology can physically remove the patient from the healthcare provider, allowing remote access to a range of healthcare services. Within this, technology enables the separation of the assessor or diagnostician of the services from the person who provides the services or manufacturer of the product. Examples include the prescription and ordering by a pedorthist of footwear that is subsequently manufactured overseas, spectacles prescribed in situ but manufactured remotely, or the remote analysis of a radiographic image. Another example is the provision of a service locally with the support of an allied health assistant who is advised or supported by a more remote 'expert', for example, the speech pathologist who advises a remote allied health assistant about the preparation of fluids for swallowing tests (Wales et al, 2017). These relationships are being tested further as artificial intelligence/machine learning improves diagnostic approaches, meaning that the relationship between the assessor and the patient will change – perhaps removing the assessor from the diagnostic relationship, or removing them from the clinical interaction altogether (Diprose and Buist, 2016; Arancibia et al, 2019). But what of the highly gendered complex and caring work? It appears that robots are even able to intervene effectively in areas of personal care (Archibald and Barnard, 2018; Melkas et al, 2020).

The 21st century will be marked by a downward pressure on costs. Disentanglement of tasks from professions is already seeing a more rapid disaggregation of roles than would have been possible or likely without a crisis situation. Where will this leave workforce roles?

Boyce has taken this concept a step further to consider 'gig-economy aggregators', in which Uber-like technology platforms offer disaggregated, on-demand allied health tasks directly to consumers

(Boyce et al, 2019). Boyce proposes that profession-led practice can be portrayed as staid and unresponsive to innovation. Instead, new, responsive models of 'service' will trump models of 'care'. The public sector may also lose workforce to the attraction of highly flexible hours offered by gig-economy businesses, a known risk in highly feminised workforces such as allied health.

Together, these innovations are reconceptualising professional monopolies over expertise and knowledge, deconstructing profession work into codifiable and commodifiable tasks, and creating a platform in which knowledge and skills can be reconstructed around the needs of the patient or client, not the traditional domains of the profession. These changes will present new challenges and opportunities for industrial relations and the regulation and safety of professional work. However, as this book illustrates, many of these changes are taking place now, within existing employment and regulatory frameworks.

Implications for the sociology of the professions

How does this study of allied health relate to the theories offered by the sociology of the professions? It remains likely that the allied health professions themselves continue to think in terms of the taxonomic approach but act in terms of the neo-Weberian approach. By this, we mean that allied health professions continue to assume that to be a professional means to act professionally, to observe and maintain standards of behaviour that fit the image of professionalism, to construe their actions as altruistic, and to promote a service ethic and orientation. It is probably fair to say that they continue to believe that their motives are not primarily economic, though those attracted to the private sector do cite high income as an incentive. There is reason to believe that their concern for the public interest is, in part, genuine, just as is the case with medicine and nursing. However, it remains abundantly clear that the professional projects of the allied health professions are actively engaged and operate continuously. Whereas some tasks may be shared willingly between groups, there remains considerable tension over how best to solve the health workforce shortages.

For the allied health professions, this reflects the need to use dual closure strategies, which, in turn, demonstrates the position they occupy in the health division of labour. They continue to seek to expand their own task domains and push back their role boundaries, while, at the same time, resisting incursions from other groups into their own core roles. They take every opportunity to flag up their skills and abilities to take on work previously exclusively medical in nature, for example, prescribing medicines, undertaking invasive surgery, acquiring qualifications in ultrasound technology and asserting their ability to make independent diagnoses, albeit in limited form. At the same time, they seek to control and regulate internally the work of support workers, aides or assistants. Thus, the explanatory power of concepts such as exclusionary and usurpationary social closure still has currency and relevance.

Jurisdictional disputes do still occur between the allied health professions or with medicine and nursing. The changing face of the healthcare workforce means that opportunities to fully engage allied health professional projects are abundant. However, they are constrained to some extent by the aims of the state as providers of most healthcare. It is clear that allied health professions continue to covet roles that were once the preserve of medicine alone, and continue to promote their advanced skills. New roles for allied health during the public health crisis presented by COVID-19 may create longer-term extensions to practice. Observed in the appropriate sociopolitical and sociohistorical context, the recent and current actions of the allied health professions continue to fit the neo-Weberian mould. Professional projects in allied health are alive and well.

Bourdieuan theory remains potent in helping to explain how professions may continue to seek to exercise power and authority, even when their ability to do so is apparently diminished. When subtly applied, the use of discursive strategies that draw upon 'doxa' – the taken-for-granted, self-evident truths – to convince key audiences can be effective. Orthopaedic surgeons' engagement with 'symbolic devaluation' continues to resonate and cast doubt on the legitimacy of those allied health practices that encroach upon their domain, even when state policy permits it, and even promotes it. Thus, even in the face of a managerialist state agenda for solving workforce shortages, medical power can be exerted and sustained, albeit in a defensive mode. This, perhaps, is also an illustration of the extent to which medical dominance, so effective during the middle part of the 20th century, has retreated in relation to allied health, and has been superseded by the interests of the state. It does not mean that the relative balance of prestige within the health division of labour has changed, or that allied health professions have gained status equivalent to medicine. Indeed, the hierarchy remains stable. Groups seeking professional status may be more easily able to achieve it, to the extent that they might swell the ranks of the allied health fold, but they do not progress beyond it, nor often seek to do so. It is a plateau that, once reached, becomes home. Thus, the allied health professions continue to grow in number but, in doing so, may be steadily losing prestige rather than gaining it. As scarcity value diminishes, and as potential competitors join the race to provide similar services, the path ahead may become harder for their professional projects.

A resurgence of interest in the technicality–indeterminacy ratio in defining the knowledge base of professions has particular relevance for the allied health professions given the way in which either they have struggled to define a sufficiently separate knowledge base from medicine, or their knowledge has been marginalised and limited. Even those allied health professions that claim to be specialists in a limited arena are often denied full jurisdiction over it because they are still unable to command the full range of activities necessary to make every diagnosis of every disorder that may occur in that domain, for example, optometrists may now prescribe medicines for common eye conditions but cannot stray very far into the domain of serious eye disease.

How, then, does this book contribute to the sociology of the professions? Perhaps it both demonstrates the ongoing relevance of sociological theory to understanding the contemporary allied health professions, and identifies areas where re-evaluation or reconsideration is timely. Having addressed the former, it may be worth considering the latter here. Perhaps the most important point is the transition in allied health from subordination to medicine, or limitation by it, to accountability to the state, and to the demands of the market, its real masters. Whether born into it (for example, radiography) or adopted by it (for example, podiatry), the dominance of the state has become more evident. Equally, the growth of independent practice in a competitive healthcare marketplace has increasingly become a key component in the overall health economy. Policy initiatives designed to address workforce shortages resulting from baby-boomer retirement and an ageing population now cast the professions in a different role. They must adapt to state demands for change, and they must serve the system rather than themselves, their worth measured by how much they alter their role to fit the needs defined from above. Private sector markets increasingly also serve state aims by providing competitive options in a neo-liberal world. Success arises from aligning with state aims. In true neo-Weberian form, what the professions seek remains constant – prestige, autonomy, social status and control. However, they do so within a new environment, born of necessity. Professions continue to compete for space, for task domains and to defend role boundaries or prestigious titles, though within a context shaped by the need to conform to political and economic solutions to healthcare workforce shortages.

Deprofessionalisation has not really occurred in the sense that the allied health professions have become increasingly necessary to the delivery of the flexible workforce required by the state. However, allied health professions have also increasingly become a commodity for use by the state, to plug gaps, to fill spaces and to be malleable in the interests of the healthcare system. In the contemporary world, allied health professions are governed by the state and market, their professional projects tailored to capitalise on opportunities arising for greater status, access to 'virtuoso' roles and greater prominence in the delivery of high-level skills. Yet, they also perhaps tailor their ambitions to fit that which is possible – the subjective expectation of objective probability, in Bourdieuan parlance. As the allied health fold becomes ever-more crowded, the allied health professions must adapt; survival may hinge on becoming what is asked of them, not what they desire.

References

Abbott, A. (1981) Status and status strain in the professions. *American Journal of Sociology* 86(4): 819–35.

Abbott, A. (1988) *The System of Professions: An Essay on the Division of Expert Labour*, Chicago, IL: University of Chicago Press.

Abbott, P. and Meerabeau, L. (1998) *The Sociology of the Caring Professions*, London: Psychology Press.

Abreu, B. C. and Peloquin, S. M. (2004) Embracing diversity in our profession. *American Journal of Occupational Therapy* 58(3): 353–9.

Abrishami, D. (2018) The need for cultural competency in health care. *Radiologic Technology* 89(5): 441–8.

ACT Health (2007) *Non-Medical Prescribing*, Canberra: ACT Health.

Adams, J. and Tochhini, L. (2015) *The Impact of Allied Health Professionals in Improving Outcomes and Reducing the Cost of Treating Diabetes, Osteoarthritis and Stroke: A Report Developed for Services for Australian Rural and Remote Allied Health*, Canberra: Services for Australian Rural and Remote Allied Health.

Adams, T. L. (1998) Combining gender, class, and race: structuring relations in the Ontario dental profession. *Gender & Society* 12(5): 578–97.

Adams, T. L. (2003) Professionalization, gender and female-dominated professions: dental hygiene in Ontario. *Canadian Review of Sociology/ Revue Canadienne de Sociologie* 40(3): 267–89.

Adams, T. L. (2004) Inter-professional conflict and professionalization: dentistry and dental hygiene in Ontario. *Social Science & Medicine* 58(11): 2243–52.

Adams, T. L. (2005) Feminization of professions: the case of women in dentistry. *Canadian Journal of Sociology/Cahiers Canadiens de Sociologie* 30(1): 71–94.

Adams, T. L. (2010) Gender and feminization in health care professions. *Sociology Compass* 4(7): 454–65.

Adams, T. L. and Bourgeault, I. L. (2004) Feminism and women's health professions in Ontario. *Women & Health* 38(4): 73–90.

Ahmed, S., Barwick, A., Butterworth, P. and Nancarrow, S. (2020) Footwear and insole design features that reduce neuropathic plantar forefoot ulcer risk in people with diabetes: a systematic literature review. *Journal of Foot and Ankle Research* 13: 1–13.

Aiken, A. B., Harrison, M. M., Atkinson, M. and Hope, J. (2008) Easing the burden for joint replacement wait times: the role of the expanded practice physiotherapist. *Healthcare Quarterly* 11(2): 62–6.

Al Busaidy, N. S. M. and Borthwick, A. (2012) Occupational therapy in Oman: the impact of cultural dissonance. *Occupational Therapy International* 19(3): 154–64.

Allen, D. (2000) Doing occupational demarcation: the 'boundary-work' of nurse managers in a district general hospital. *Journal of Contemporary Ethnography* 29(3): 326–56.

Allen, N. A. (2003) The history of diabetes nursing, 1914–1936. *The Diabetes Educator* 29(6): 976–89.

Allied Health Aotearoa New Zealand (no date) Become a member, www.alliedhealth.org.nz/membership.html

Allied Health Professions Australia (no date) Become a member, https://ahpa.com.au/become-a-member/

Allsop, J. and Saks, M. (2003) *Regulating the Health Professions*, London: Sage.

Andrews, G. J. and Evans, J. (2008) Understanding the reproduction of health care: towards geographies in health care work. *Progress in Human Geography* 32(6): 759–80.

Antwi, W. K., Kyei, K. A. and Quarcoopome, L. N. (2014) Effectiveness of multicultural communication between radiographers and patients and its impact on outcome of examinations. *World Journal of Medical Research* 3(4).

Arancibia, J. N., Sánchez, F. J. M., Del Rey Mejías, Á., Del Castillo, J. G., Cháfer, J., Briñon, M. G., Cadenas, M. S., Mayol, J. and Aguilar, G. S. (2019) Evaluation of a diagnostic decision support system for the triage of patients in a hospital emergency department. *International Journal of Interactive Multimedia and Artificial Intelligence* 5(4): 60–7.

Archibald, M. M. and Barnard, A. (2018) Futurism in nursing: technology, robotics and the fundamentals of care. *Journal of Clinical Nursing* 27(11/12): 2473–80.

Arsenault, P. R. (2000) The role of the perfusionist. *Journal of Infusion Nursing* 23(2): 99–104.

Atkinson, K. (1993) Reprofiling and skill mix: our next challenge. *British Journal of Occupational Therapy* 56(2): 67–9.

Australian Diabetes Educators Association (2015a) Annual report 2014–15, www.adea.com.au/wp-content/uploads/2016/09/Annual-Report-2015-final-web-12082015.pdf

Australian Diabetes Educators Association (2015b) *Information for Preparing Your Application: Initial Credentialling*, Canberra, Australia: Australian Diabetes Educators Association.

Australian Government (2020) *Commonwealth Home Support Programme*, Canberra: Australian Government.

Australian Health Ministers' Advisory Council (2018) Information on regulatory assessment criteria and process for adding new professions to the National Registration and Accreditation Scheme for the health professions. AHMAC.

Australian Health Workforce Advisory Committee (2006) *The Australian Allied Health Workforce: An Overview of Workforce Planning Issues*, Sydney: AHWAC Report 2006, 1.

Awaad, J. (2003) Culture, cultural competency and occupational therapy: a review of the literature. *British Journal of Occupational Therapy* 66(8): 356–62.

Bach, S., Kessler, I. and Heron, P. (2008) Role redesign in a modernised NHS: the case of health care assistants. *Human Resource Management Journal* 18(2): 171–87.

Bacon, D. and Borthwick, A. M. (2013) Charismatic authority in modern healthcare: the case of the 'diabetes specialist podiatrist'. *Sociology of Health & Illness* 35(7): 1080–94.

Baer, H. A. (2009) Osteopathy in Australasia: from marginality to a fully professionalised system of health care. *International Journal of Osteopathic Medicine* 12(1): 25–31.

Barber, B. (1963) Some problems in the sociology of professions. *Daedalus* 92: 669–88.

Bashshur, R., Doarn, C. R., Frenk, J. M., Kvedar, J. C. and Woolliscroft, J. O. (2020) *Telemedicine and the COVID-19 Pandemic, Lessons for the Future*, New York, NY: Mary Ann Liebert, Inc.

Beech, J., Bottery, S., Charlesworth, A., Evans, H., Gershlick, B., Hemmings, N., Imison, C., Kahtan, P., McKenna, H. and Murray, R. (2019) *Closing the Gap: Key Areas for Action on the Health and Care Workforce*, London: Kings Fund.

Bennett, C. J. and Grant, M. J. (2004) Specialisation in physiotherapy: a mark of maturity. *Australian Journal of Physiotherapy* 50(1): 3–5.

Berlant, J. L. (1975) *Profession and Monopoly: A Study of Medicine in the United States and Great Britain*, Berkeley, CA: University of California Press.

Berwick, D. M. (2003) Improvement, trust, and the healthcare workforce. *BMJ Quality & Safety* 12(6): 448–52.

Bishu, S. G., Guy, M. E. and Heckler, N. (2019) Seeing gender and its consequences. *Journal of Public Affairs Education* 25(2): 145–62.

Black, R. M. (2002) Occupational therapy's dance with diversity. *American Journal of Occupational Therapy* 56(2): 140–8.

Bochatay, N. (2018) Individual and collective strategies in nurses' struggle for professional identity. *Health Sociology Review* 27(1): 1–16.

Boden, I., Skinner, E. H., Browning, L., Reeve, J., Anderson, L., Hill, C., Robertson, I. K., Story, D. and Denehy, L. (2018) Preoperative physiotherapy for the prevention of respiratory complications after upper abdominal surgery: pragmatic, double blinded, multicentre randomised controlled trial. *British Medical Journal* 360: j5916.

Boniol, M., McIsaac, M., Xu, L., Wuliji, T., Diallo, K. and Campbell, J. (2019) *Gender Equity in the Health Workforce: Analysis of 104 Countries*, Geneva: World Health Organization.

Boreham, P. (1983) Indetermination: professional knowledge, organisation and control. *Sociological Review* 31(4): 693–718.

Borthwick, A. (1999) Perspectives on podiatric biomechanics: Foucault and the professional project. *British Journal of Podiatry* 2(1): 21–8.

Borthwick, A. (2000) Challenging medicine: the case of podiatric surgery. *Work, Employment and Society* 14(2): 369–83.

Borthwick, A. (2001a) Drug prescribing in podiatry: radicalism or tokenism? *British Journal of Podiatry* 4(2): 56–64.

Borthwick, A. (2001b) Occupational imperialism at work: the case of podiatric surgery. *British Journal of Podiatry* 4(3): 70–9.

Borthwick, A. (2005) 'In the beginning': local anaesthesia and the Croydon Postgraduate Group. *British Journal of Podiatry* 8(3): 87–94.

Borthwick, A. (2008) Professions allied to medicine and prescribing. In: Nolan, P. and Bradley, E. (eds) *Non-Medical Prescribing – Multi-Disciplinary Perspectives*, Cambridge: Cambridge University Press.

Borthwick, A., Boyce, R. A. and Nancarrow, S. A. (2015) Symbolic power and professional titles: the case of 'podiatric surgery'. *Health Sociology Review* 24(3): 310–22.

Borthwick, A., Nancarrow, S. A., Vernon, W. and Walker, J. (2009) Achieving professional status: Australian podiatrists' perceptions. *Journal of Foot and Ankle Research* 2(1): 4.

Borthwick, A., Short, A., Nancarrow, S. and Boyce, R. (2010) Non-medical prescribing in Australasia and the UK: the case of podiatry. *Journal of Foot and Ankle Research* 3(1).

Borthwick, A., Kilmartin, T., Freeman, C. and Wilson, N. (2017) Allied health prescribing. In: Franklin, P. (ed) *Non-Medical Prescribing in the UK*, London: Springer.

Bourdieu, P. (1985) The social space and the genesis of groups. *Theory and Society* 14(6): 723–7.

Bourdieu, P. and Passeron, J. C. (1990) *Reproduction in Education, Society and Culture*, London: Sage.

Bourgeault, I. L., Maier, C. B., Dieleman, M., Ball, J., Mackenzie, A., Nancarrow, S., Nigenda, G. and Sidat, M. (2020) The COVID-19 pandemic presents an opportunity to develop more sustainable health workforces. *Human Resources for Health* 18(1): 1–8.

Boyce, R. (1996) The organisation of allied health professions in Australian general hospitals. PhD thesis, School of Management, QUT.

Boyce, R. (2001) Organisational governance structures in allied health services: a decade of change. *Australian Health Review* 24(1): 22–36.

Boyce, R. (2006) Emerging from the shadow of medicine: allied health as a 'profession community' subculture. *Health Sociology Review* 15(5): 520–34.

Boyce, R. and Jackway, P. (2016) Allied health leaders: Australian public sector health boards and top management teams. Victorian Department of Health and Human Services, Office of the Chief Allied Health Advisor.

Boyce, R., Nancarrow, S. A., King, O. and Jackway, P. (2019) *Retrospective Analysis and Future Trends in Allied Health Leadership and Workforce: From Therapy Divisions to Gig-Economy Aggregators. 13th National Allied Health Conference.* Brisbane, Australia: Allied Health Professions Australia.

Boyd, S. and Hewlett, N. (2001) The gender imbalance among speech and language therapists and students. *International Journal of Language & Communication Disorders* 36(S1): 167–72.

Bradd, P., Travaglia, J. and Hayen, A. (2018) Allied health leadership in New South Wales: a study of perceptions and priorities of allied health leaders. *Australian Health Review* 42(3): 316–20.

Braverman, H. (1974) *Labour and Monopoly Capital: The Degradation of Work in the Twentieth Century*, New York, NY: Monthly Review Press.

British Medical Association (ed.) (2020) *Speciality Explorer*, London: BMA.

Brooks, C., Ballinger, C., Nutbeam, D., Mander, C. and Adams, J. (2020) Nursing and allied health professionals' views about using health literacy screening tools and a universal precautions approach to communication with older adults: a qualitative study. *Disability and Rehabilitation* 42(13): 1819–25.

Brusin, J. H. (2012) How cultural competency can help reduce health disparities. *Radiologic Technology* 84(2): 129–52.

Buchan, J. and Dal Poz, M. R. (2002) Skill mix in the health care workforce: reviewing the evidence. *Bulletin of the World Health Organization* 80(7): 575–80.

Buckmaster, L. and Clark, S. (2018) The National Disability Insurance Scheme: a chronology. Department of Parliamentary Services, Parliamentary Library.

Buss, V. H., Deeks, L. S., Shield, A., Kosari, S. and Naunton, M. (2019) Analytical quality and effectiveness of point-of-care testing in community pharmacies: a systematic literature review. *Research in Social and Administrative Pharmacy* 15(5): 483–95.

Butteriss, M. A. (2012) NDIS: in context. *Journal of Social Inclusion* 3(2): 102–7.

Cameron, A. and Masterson, A. (2003) Reconfiguring the clinical workforce. In: Davies, C. (ed) *The Future Health Workforce*, Basingstoke: Palgrave Macmillan.

Canadian Medical Association (2020) Canadian speciality profiles, www.cma.ca/canadian-specialty-profiles

Cant, R. P. and Foster, M. M. (2011) Investing in big ideas: utilisation and cost of Medicare Allied Health services in Australia under the Chronic Disease Management initiative in primary care. *Australian Health Review* 35(4): 468–74.

Carchedi, G. (1975) On the economic identification of the new middle class. *Economy and Society* 4(1): 1–86.

Carey, G., Malbon, E., Green, C., Reeders, D. and Marjolin, A. (2020) Quasi-market shaping, stewarding and steering in personalization: the need for practice-orientated empirical evidence. *Policy Design and Practice* 3(1): 30-44.

Carlton, A.-L. (2017) The forces shaping regulation of the health professions in Australia: from 'club government' to inclusive regulatory institutions. PhD thesis, Latrobe University.

Carmel, S. (2006) Boundaries obscured and boundaries reinforced: incorporation as a strategy of occupational enhancement for intensive care. *Sociology of Health & Illness* 28(2): 154–77.

Carpenter, E. S. (1977) Women in male-dominated health professions. *International Journal of Health Services* 7(2): 191–207.

Carr-Saunders, A. and Wilson, P. (1933) *The Professions*, London: Frank Cass and Company.

Carvalho, T. (2014) Changing connections between professionalism and managerialism: a case study of nursing in Portugal. *Journal of Professions and Organization* 1(2): 176–90.

Cathrael Kazin, J. and Clerkin, K. M. (2018) The potential and limitations of microcredentials, http://supportsystem.livehelpnow. net/resources/23351/Potential%20and%20Limitations%20of%20 Microcredentials%20FINAL_SEPT%202018.pdf

Cena, L., McGruder, J. and Tomlin, G. (2002) Representations of race, ethnicity, and social class in case examples in *The American Journal of Occupational Therapy*. *American Journal of Occupational Therapy* 56(2): 130–9.

Chamberlain, J. (2015) *Medical Regulation, Fitness to Practice and Medical Revalidation: A Critical Introduction*, Bristol: Policy Press.

Chamberlain, J. (2018) Introduction: professional health regulation in the public interest. In: Chamberlain, J., Dent, M. and Saks, M. (eds) *Professional Health Regulation in the Public Interest*, Bristol: Policy Press.

Changing Workforce Programme (2003) *Developing Support Worker Roles in Rehabilitation in Intermediate Care Services*, London: National Health Service.

Chau, M. (2020) Cultural diversity and the importance of communication, cultural competence, and uncertainty in radiography. *Journal of Medical Imaging and Radiation Sciences*, DOI: https://doi.org/10.1016/j.jmir.2020.04.005

Chen, M.-S. (2001) *The Great Reversal: Transformation of Health Care in the People's Republic of China*. In: Cockerham, W. C. (ed) *The Blackwell Companion to Medical Sociology*, Oxford: Blackwell Publishers, 456–482.

Chipchase, L. S., Jull, P., McMeeken, J., Refshauge, K., Nayler, M. and Wright, A. (2006) Looking back at 100 years of physiotherapy education in Australia. *Australian Journal of Physiotherapy* 52(1): 3.

Cole, B. L. (2015a) *A History of Australian Optometry: Two Hundred Years of Beating the Tyranny of Distance and Fighting Political Battles to Find New Roles and a New Place in Health Care*, Melbourne, Australia: Australian College of Optometry.

Cole, B. L. (2015b) A short history of the Australian College of Optometry 1940–2015. *Clinical and Experimental Optometry* 98(5): 411–19.

College of Occupational Therapists (1993) *Position Statement on Skill Mix in the NHS and Its Implications for Occupational Therapy Staff*, London: COT.

College of Podiatry (2020) Assistant practitioners, College of Podiatrists, https://cop.org.uk/events-and-courses/assistant-practitioner-training

Collins, R. (1990a) *Changing Conceptions in the Sociology of the Professions*, London: Sage.

Collins, R. (1990b) Market closure and the conflict theory of the professions. In: Burrage, W. and Torstendahl, R. (eds) *Professions in Theory and History*. London: Sage.

Commissioner for Public Sector Employment (2011) Public Sector Act 2009, Adelaide: Government of South Australia.

Cook, T., Kursumovic, E. and Lennane, S. (2020) Exclusive: deaths of NHS staff from covid-19 analysed. *Health Service Journal* 22, www.hsj.co.uk/exclusive-deaths-of-nhs-staff-from-covid-19-analysed/7027471.article

Copnell, G. (2010) Modernising allied health professions careers: attacking the foundations of the professions? *Journal of Interprofessional Care* 24(1): 63–9.

Corbett, R. and Suckling, S. (2018) Professionalisation of operating department practice: an evolutionary perspective. *Journal of Education and Work* 31(4): 381–93.

Coulter, I. and Willis, E. (2007) Explaining the growth of complementary and alternative medicine. *Health Sociology Review* 16(3/4): 214–25.

Courtenay, M., Nancarrow, S. and Dawson, D. (2013) Interprofessional teamwork in the trauma setting: a scoping review. *Human Resources for Health* 11(1): 57.

Cox, D. (1991) Health service management – a sociological view: Griffiths and the non-negotiated order of the hospital. In: Gabe, J., Calnan, M. and Bury, M. (eds) *The Sociology of the Health Service*, London: Routledge.

Currie, G., Finn, R. and Martin, G. (2009) Professional competition and modernizing the clinical workforce in the NHS. *Work, Employment & Society* 23(2): 267–84.

Cuthbert, M. (2013) *Q&A European Union Law 2013–2014*, London: Routledge.

Dagnall, J. (1983) A history of chiropody–podiatry and foot care. *British Journal of Chiropody* 48(7): 137–83.

Dagnall, J. (1995a) The origins of the Society of Chiropodists and Podiatrists and its history 1945–1995 (part 1). *Journal of British Podiatric Medicine* 50(9): 135–41.

Dagnall, J. (1995b) The origins of the Society of Chiropodists and Podiatrists 1945–1995 (part 2). *Journal of British Podiatric Medicine* 50(10): 151–6.

Dagnall, J. (1995c) The origins of the Society of Chiropodists and Podiatrists 1945–1995 (part 3). *Journal of British Podiatric Medicine* 50(11): 174–80.

Dahl-Michelsen, T. (2014) Sportiness and masculinities among female and male physiotherapy students. *Physiotherapy Theory and Practice* 30(5): 329–37.

Dahl-Michelsen, T. and Leseth, A. (2011) Treningskultur og profesjonsidentitet i en norsk fysioterapeututdanning. In: Leseth, A. and Solbrække, K.N. (eds) *Profesjon, Kjønn og Etnisitet*, Oslo: Cappelen Damm.

Dahl-Michelsen, T. and Solbrække, K.N. (2014) When bodies matter: significance of the body in gender constructions in physiotherapy education. *Gender and Education* 26(6), 672–87.

Davies, M. (1985) *The Essential Social Worker*, Aldershot: Gower.

Dawber, J., Crow, N., Hulcombe, J. and Mickan, S. (2017) A realist review of allied health management in Queensland Health: what works, in which contexts and why, Queensland Health, Queensland Government, www.health.qld.gov.au/__data/assets/pdf_file/0024/691431/ah-mgmt-in-qh.pdf

Dent, M. and Whitehead, S. (2002) *Managing Professional Identities: Knowledge, Performativity and the 'New' Professional*, London: Routledge.

Dent, M., Chandler, J. and Barry, J. (2004) Introduction: questioning the new public management. In: Dent, M., Chandler, J. and Barry, J. (eds) *Questioning the New Public Management*, London: Routledge.

Department of Health (1994) *Feet First: Report of the Joint Department of Health and NHS Chiropody Task Force*, London: HMSO.

Department of Health (1999) *Final Report of the Review of Prescribing, Supply and Administration of Medicines (Crown Report)*, London: Department of Health.

Department of Health (2000) *Meeting the Challenge: A Strategy for the Allied Health Professions*, London: Department for Health.

Department of Health (2001) *Agenda for Change*, London: Department of Health.

Department of Health (2002) *HR in the NHS Plan: More Staff Working Differently*, London: Department of Health.

Department of Health (2004a) *Agenda for Change: What Will It Mean for You? A Guide for Staff*, London: Department of Health.

Department of Health (2004b) *Executive Letter 02/12/2004: Implementation of Agenda for Change from 1st December 2004*, London: Department of Health.

Department of Health (2004c) *The NHS Knowledge and Skills Framework (NHS KSF) and the Development Review Process*, London: Department of Health.

Department of Health (2009) *Allied Health Professions, Prescribing and Medicines Supply Scoping Project Report*, London: Department of Health.

Developmental Educators Australia Incorporated (2020) Home page, www.deai.com.au/

Diprose, W. and Buist, N. (2016) Artificial intelligence in medicine: humans need not apply? *The New Zealand Medical Journal (Online)* 129(1434): 73.

Donini-Lenhoff, F. G. and Brotherton, S. E. (2010) Racial-ethnic diversity in allied health: the continuing challenge. *Journal of Allied Health* 39(2): 104–9.

Doyal, L. (1979) *The Political Economy of Health*, London: Pluto Press.

Duckett, S. (2005) Health workforce design for the 21st century. *Australian Health Review* 29(2): 201–10.

Dwairy, M. and Van Sickle, T. D. (1996) Western psychotherapy in traditional Arabic societies. *Clinical Psychology Review* 16(3): 231–49.

Editorial (1989) Footcare assistants. *The Chiropodist* 44(12): 265.

Editorial (1999) International podiatry. *British Journal of Podiatry* 3(4): 34.

Editorial (2000) International qualifications. *British Journal of Podiatry* 3(4): 90.

Ehrenreich, B. and Ehrenreich, J. (1979) The professional–managerial class. In: Walker, P. (ed) *Between Labor and Capital*, Boston, MA: South End Press.

Ellison, C. and Matthews, B. (2012) Disability professionals: assisting people living with disability to navigate the health system. In: Willis, E., Reynolds, L. and Keleher, H. (eds) *Understanding the Australian Health Care System*, Sydney: Churchill Livingstone.

Elston, M. (1991) The politics of professional power: medicine in a changing health service. In: Gabe, J., Calnan, M. and Bury, M. (eds) *The Sociology of the Health Service*, London: Routledge.

Emerson, E. and McGill, P. (1989) Normalization and applied behaviour analysis: values and technology in services for people with learning difficulties. *Behavioural and Cognitive Psychotherapy* 17(2): 101–17.

Enoch, J. M. (2006) History of mirrors dating back 8000 years. *Optometry and Vision Science* 83(10): 775–81.

Eribon, D. (1992) *Michel Foucault*, Cambridge: Harvard University Press.

Esland, G. (1980) Professions and professionalism. In: Esland, G. and Salaman, G. (eds) *The Politics of Work and Occupations*, Milton Keynes: Open University Press.

Etzioni, A. (1969) *The Semi-Professions and Their Organization: Teachers, Nurses, Social Workers*, New York: Free Press.

Evans, J. (1992) What occupational therapists can do to eliminate racial barriers to health care access. *American Journal of Occupational Therapy* 46(8): 679–83.

Evetts, J. (2011) A new professionalism? Challenges and opportunities. *Current Sociology* 59(4): 406–22.

Exworthy, M. and Halford, S. (1999) *Professionals and New Managerialism in the Public Sector*, Buckingham: Open University Press.

Farndon, L. and Nancarrow, S. (2003) Employment and career development opportunities for podiatrists and foot care assistants in the NHS. *British Journal of Podiatry* 6(4): 103–8.

Farndon, L., Vernon, W. and Parry, A. (2006) What is the evidence for the continuation of core podiatry services in the National Health Service: a review of foot surveys? *Australasian Journal of Podiatric Medicine* 40(2): 35.

Finn, R. (2008) The language of teamwork: reproducing professional divisions in the operating theatre. *Human Relations* 61(1): 103–30.

Flynn, R. (1999) Managerialism, professionalism and quasi-markets. In: Exworthy, M. and Halford, S. (eds) *Professionals and the New Managerialism in the Public Sector*, Buckingham: Open University Press.

Foo, J. S., Storr, M. and Maloney, S. (2016) Registration factors that limit international mobility of people holding physiotherapy qualifications: a systematic review. *Health Policy* 120(6): 665–73.

Foucault, M. (1979) *Discipline and Punish*, London: Penguin.

Francis, B. (1999) Rationalisation and professionalisation: a comparison of the transfer of registered nurse education to higher education in Australia and the UK. *Comparative Education* 35(1): 81–96.

Francis, G. and Hogg, D. (2006) Radiographer prescribing: enhancing seamless care in oncology. *Radiography* 12: 3–5.

Freidson, E. (1970) *Professional Dominance: The Social Structure of Medical Care*, New York, NY: Atherton Press.

Freidson, E. (1988) *Profession of Medicine: A Study of the Sociology of Applied Knowledge*, London: University of Chicago Press.

Freidson, E. (1994) *Professionalism Reborn: Theory, Prophecy and Policy*, Cambridge: Polity Press.

Freidson, E. (2001) *Professionalism: The Third Logic*, Oxford: Oxford University Press.

Gardner, G., Duffield, C., Doubrovsky, A. and Adams, M. (2016) Identifying advanced practice: a national survey of a nursing workforce. *International Journal of Nursing Studies* 55: 60–70.

George, K. and George, G. (2014) Intellectual Disabilities Services Council (1976–2006). Find and Connect, www.findandconnect.gov. au/ref/sa/biogs/SE01312b.htm

Gilheany, M. and Borthwick, A. (2009) Recent developments in podiatric prescribing in the UK and Australia. *Journal of Foot and Ankle Research* 2: 37.

Godin, P. (1996) The development of community psychiatric nursing: a professional project? *Journal of Advanced Nursing* 23(5): 925–34.

Graham, M. (2006) The origins and development of podiatry in Britain 1969–1996. PhD thesis, University of Essex.

Gray, M., Thomas, Y., Bonassi, M., Elston, J. and Tapia, G. (2020) Cultural safety training for allied health students in Australia. *The Australian Journal of Indigenous Education*, http://eprints.worc.ac.uk/9440/

Greenwood, N. and Bithell, C. (2005) Perceptions of physiotherapy compared with nursing and medicine amongst minority ethnic and white UK students: implications for recruitment. *Physiotherapy* 91(2): 69–78.

Greenwood, N., Wright, J. A. and Bithell, C. (2006) Perceptions of speech and language therapy amongst UK school and college students: implications for recruitment. *International Journal of Language & Communication Disorders* 41(1): 83–94.

Grumbach, K. and Mendoza, R. (2008) Disparities in human resources: addressing the lack of diversity in the health professions. *Health Affairs* 27(2): 413–22.

Ham, C. (2004) *Health Policy in Britain*, Basingstoke: Palgrave Macmillan.

Hambleton, S. (2012) Hands off prescribing. *Australian Medicine* 24: 3.

Hamilton, J. (2011) Two birds with one stone: addressing interprofessional education aims and objectives in health profession curricula through interdisciplinary cultural competency training. *Medical Teacher* 33(4): e199–e203.

Hammond, J. A. (2009) Assessment of clinical components of physiotherapy undergraduate education: are there any issues with gender? *Physiotherapy* 95(4): 266–72.

Hammond, J. A., Williams, A., Walker, S. and Norris, M. (2019) Working hard to belong: a qualitative study exploring students from black, Asian and minority ethnic backgrounds experiences of pre-registration physiotherapy education. *BMC Medical Education* 19(1): 1–11.

Han, E. (2018) NSW Premier rejects nurses' demand for higher nurse-to-patient ratios. *Sydney Morning Herald*, 18 September.

Hancock, H., Campbell, S., Ramprogus, V. and Kilgour, J. (2005) Role development in health care assistants: the impact of education on practice. *Journal of Evaluation in Clinical Practice* 11(5): 489–98.

Haralambos, M. and Holborn, M. (2008) *Sociology: Themes and Perspectives*, London: HarperCollins UK.

Hardy, M. L., Legg, J., Smith, T., Ween, B., Williams, I. and Motto, J. (2008) The concept of advance radiographic practice: an international perspective. *Radiography* (14): e14–e19.

Harrits, G. S. (2014) Professional closure beyond state authorization. *Professions and Professionalism* 4(1): 1–17.

Harvey-Lloyd, J. and Strudwick, R. (2018) Embracing diversity in radiography: the role of service users. *Radiography* 24: S16–S19.

Hassall, L. (2007) Sonography – the emergence of a profession. *ASUM Ultrasound Bulletin* 10(3): 29–34.

Haug, M. R. (1975) The deprofessionalization of everyone? *Sociological Focus* 8(3): 197–213.

Health Care Professions Council (no date) Standards, www.hcpc-uk.org/standards/

Health Professions Council of Australia (1998) Membership brochure. Health Professions Council of Australia.

Healy, E., Kiely, P. M. and Arunachalam, D. (2015) Optometric supply and demand in Australia: 2011–2036. *Clinical and Experimental Optometry* 98(3): 273–82.

Heap, R. (1995) Physiotherapy's quest for professional status in Ontario, 1950–80. *Canadian Bulletin of Medical History* 12(1): 69–99.

Hill-Briggs, F., Kelly, K. and Ewing, C. (2010) Challenges to providing culturally competent care in medical rehabilitation to African Americans. In: Balcazar, F., Suarez-Balcazar, Y., Taylor-Ritzler, T. and Keys, C. (eds) *Race, Culture, and Disability: Rehabilitation Science and Practice*, Sudbury, MA: Jones and Bartlett.

Hilless, M., Healy, J. and World Health Organization (2001) *Health Care Systems In Transition: Australia*, Copenhagen: WHO Regional Office for Europe.

Hirama, H. (1994) Should certified occupational therapy assistants provide occupational therapy services independently? *American Journal of Occupational Therapy* 48(9): 840–3.

Hogg, P. and Hogg, D. (2003) Radiographer prescribing: lessons to be learnt from the community nursing experience. *Radiography* 9: 263–5.

Hogg, P., Francis, G., Mountain, V., Pitt, A., Sherrington, S. and Freeman, C. (2007) Prescription, supply and administration of medicines in radiography: current position and future directions. *Synergy News – Imaging and Therapy Practice* December: 26–31.

Howe, D. (1986) *Social Workers and Their Practice in Welfare Bureaucracies*, Aldershot: Gower.

Hsieh, C.-R. and Tang, C. (2019) The multi-tiered medical education system and its influence on the health care market: China's Flexner Report. *Human Resources for Health* 17(1): 50.

Hu, D., Zhu, W., Fu, Y., Zhang, M., Zhao, Y., Hanson, K., Martinez-Alvarez, M. and Liu, X. (2017) Development of village doctors in China: financial compensation and health system support. *International Journal for Equity in Health* 16(1): 9.

Hugman, R. (1991) *Power in the Caring Professions*, Basingstoke: Macmillan.

Jaggi, A. and Bithell, C. (1995) Relationships between physiotherapists' level of contact, cultural awareness and communication with Bangladeshi patients in two health authorities. *Physiotherapy* 81(6): 330–7.

Jamous, H. and Peloille, B. (1970) Professions or self-perpetuating system: changes in French university hospital system. In: Jackson, J. A. (ed) *Professions and Professionalization*, Cambridge: Cambridge University Press.

Jenkins, R. (2002) *Pierre Bourdieu*, London: Routledge.

Jerjes, W. (2011) Use of medical titles by non-doctors can mislead patients. *British Medical Journal* 343: d4241.

Johnson, T. (1977) The professions in the class structure. In: Scase, R. (ed) *Industrial Class, Cleavage and Control*, London: Allen and Unwin.

Johnson, T. (1993) Expertise and the state. In: Gane, M. and Johnston, T. (eds) *Foucault's New Domains*, London: Routledge.

Kelly, J., Hogg, P. and Henwood, S. (2008) The role of a consultant breast radiographer: a description and a reflection. *Radiography* 14: e2–e10.

Kennedy, S. (2002) Explaining gender divisions of labour in physiotherapy and radiography: a qualitative study. PhD thesis, University of Sheffield.

King, O. (2018) Role boundaries and scopes of practice: the interdisciplinary diabetes educator role. PhD thesis, Southern Cross University.

King, O., Nancarrow, S. A., Borthwick, A. M. and Grace, S. (2015) Contested professional role boundaries in health care: a systematic review of the literature. *Journal of Foot and Ankle Research* 8(1): 1–9.

King, O., Nancarrow, S., Grace, S. and Borthwick, A. (2017a) Diabetes educator role boundaries: a documentary analysis. *Journal of Foot and Ankle Research*, DOI 10.1186/s13047-017-0210-9

King, R., Tod, A. and Sanders, T. (2017b) Development and regulation of advanced nurse practitioners in the UK and internationally. *Nursing Standard* 32(14): 43–50.

King, O., Borthwick, A., Nancarrow, S. and Grace, S. (2018) Sociology of the professions: what it means for podiatry. *Journal of Foot and Ankle Research* 11(30).

King, O., Nancarrow, S., Grace, S. and Borthwick, A. (2019) Interprofessional role boundaries in diabetes education in Australia. *Health Sociology Review* 28(2): 1–15.

Kings Fund (2014) *The UK Private Health Market*, London: Kings Fund.

Komaric, N., Bedford, S. and Van Driel, M. L. (2012) Two sides of the coin: patient and provider perceptions of health care delivery to patients from culturally and linguistically diverse backgrounds. *BMC Health Services Research* 12(1): 322.

Konstantakopoulou, E., Harper, R. A., Edgar, D. F., Larkin, G., Janikoun, S. and Lawrenson J. G. (2018) Clinical safety of a minor eye conditions scheme in England delivered by community optometrists. *BMJ Open Ophthalmology* 3: e000125, DOI:10.1136/bmjophth-2017-000125

Kreindler, S. A., Dowd, D. A., Dana Star, N. and Gottschalk, T. (2012) Silos and social identity: the social identity approach as a framework for understanding and overcoming divisions in health care. *The Milbank Quarterly* 90(2): 347–74.

Kritzer, H. M. (1999) The professions are dead, long live the professions: legal practice in a postprofessional world. *Law & Society Review* 33: 713.

Kuhlmann, E. and Saks, M. (2008) *Rethinking Professional Governance: International Directions in Healthcare*, Bristol: Policy Press.

Lai, G. C., Taylor, E. V., Haigh, M. M. and Thompson, S. C. (2018) Factors affecting the retention of indigenous Australians in the health workforce: a systematic review. *International Journal of Environmental Research and Public Health* 15(5): 914.

Laing, P., Ribbans, B., Parsons, S. and Winson, I. (2007) *BOFAS Business Plan for Development of Foot and Ankle Surgery with Podiatry*, London: British Orthopaedic Foot and Ankle Society.

Larkin, G. V. (1981) Professional autonomy and the opthalmic optician. *Sociology of Health and Illness* 3(1): 15–30.

Larkin, G. V. (1983) *Occupational Monopoly and Modern Medicine*, London: Tavistock.

Larkin, G. V. (2002) The regulation of the professions allied to medicine. In: Allsop, J. and Saks, M. (eds) *Regulating the Health Professions*, London: SAGE.

Larsen, Ø. and Hodne, F. (1988) Health conditions, population and physicians in Norway 1814–1986: Notes on the development of a profession. In: Brandstrom, A. and Tedebrand, L. (eds) *Society, Health and Population during the Demographic Transition*, Stockholm: Almqvist and Wiskell International.

Larson, M. (1977) *The Rise of Professionalism: A Sociological Analysis*, London: University of California Press.

Larson, M. (1990) On the matter of experts and professional, or how it is impossible to leave nothing unsaid. In: Torstendahl, R. and Burrage, M. (eds) *The Formation of Professions: Knowledge, State and Strategy*, London: Sage.

Le Cornu, K., Halliday, D., Swift, L., Ferris, L. and Gatiss, G. (2010) The current and future role of the dietetic support worker. *Journal of Human Nutrition and Dietetics* 23(3): 230–7.

Leicht, K. and Fennell, M. L. (2001) *Professional Work: A Sociological Approach*, Oxford: Blackwell Publishers.

Lester, S. (2016) The development of self-regulation in four UK professional communities. *Professions and Professionalism* 6(1), DOI: https://doi.org/10.7577/pp.1441

Lewis, S. J. (2003) Ethics and the professional status of radiography in Australia: a qualitative comparison of Australian and United Kingdom radiographers. PhD thesis, University of Sydney.

Lindsay, S. (2005) The feminization of the physician assistant profession. *Women & Health* 41(4): 37–61.

Linker, B. (2005) The business of ethics: gender, medicine, and the professional codification of the American Physiotherapy Association, 1918–1935. *Journal of the History of Medicine and Allied Sciences* 60(3): 320–54.

Littler, C. R. (1978) Understanding Taylorism. *British Journal of Sociology* 29(2): 185–202.

Lizarondo, L., Kumar, S., Hyde, L. and Skidmore, D. (2010) Allied health assistants and what they do: a systematic review of the literature. *Journal of Multidisciplinary Healthcare* 3: 143.

Long, A. F., Kneafsey, R., Ryan, J. and Berry, J. (2002) The role of the nurse within the multi-professional rehabilitation team. *Journal of Advanced Nursing* 37(1): 70–8.

Macdonald, K. M. (1995) *The Sociology of the Professions*, London: SAGE Publications.

MacDonald, R. and Rowe, N. (1995) Minority ethnic groups and occupational therapy, part 2: transcultural occupational therapy, a curriculum for today's therapist. *British Journal of Occupational Therapy* 58(7): 286–90.

Mackey, H. (2007) "Do not ask me to remain the same": Foucault and the professional identities of occupational therapists. *Australian Occupational Therapy Journal* 54(2): 95–102.

Mackey, H. and Nancarrow, S. (2004) Report on the introduction and evaluation of an assistant practitioner in occupational therapy. Shropshire & Staffordshire Workforce Development Confederation.

Mackey, H. and Nancarrow, S. (2005) Assistant practitioners: issues of accountability, delegation and competence. *International Journal of Therapy and Rehabilitation* 12(8): 331–8.

Maclean, V. M. and Rozier, C. (2009) From sport culture to the social world of the 'good PT': masculinities and the career development of physical therapists. *Men and Masculinities* 11(3): 286–306.

Maldonado, L. E. and Huda, K. (2018) Increasing the cultural competence of student radiographers. *Radiologic Technology* 89(6): 616–20.

Malin, N., Wilmot, S. and Manthorpe, J. (2002) *Key Concepts and Debates in Health and Social Care*, Maidenhead: Open University Press.

Mason, C. and Sparkes, V. J. (2002) Widening participation in physiotherapy education: part 2: ethnicity among undergraduates. *Physiotherapy* 88(5): 276–84.

Mason, J. (2013) *Review of Australian Government Health Workforce Programs*, Canberra, Australia: Australian Government.

Mavromaras, K., Moskos, M., Mahuteau, S., Isherwood, L., Goode, A., Walton, H., Smith, L., Wei, Z. and Flavel, J. (2018) *Evaluation of the NDIS. Final report*, Adelaide: National Institute of Labour Studies, Flinders University.

McBride, L.-J., Fitzgerald, C., Costello, C. and Perkins, K. (2018) Allied health pre-entry student clinical placement capacity: can it be sustained? *Australian Health Review* 44: 39–46.

McClimens, A., Nancarrow, S., Moran, A., Enderby, P. and Mitchell, C. (2010) 'Riding the bumpy seas': or the impact of the knowledge skills framework component of the Agenda for Change initiative on staff in intermediate care settings. *Journal of Interprofessional Care* 24(1): 70–9.

McComas, J., Hébert, C., Giacomin, C., Kaplan, D. and Dulberg, C. (1993) Experiences of student and practicing physical therapists with inappropriate patient sexual behavior. *Physical Therapy* 73(11): 762–9.

McKinlay, J. and Arches, J. (1985) Towards the proletarianization of physicians. *International Journal of Health Services* 18: 161–95.

McPherson, K., Kersten, P., George, S., Lattimer, V., Ellis, B., Breton, A., Kaur, D. and Frampton, G. (2004) *Extended Roles for Allied Health Professionals in the NHS.* London: NHS Service and Delivery Organisations (SDO).

Medical Board of Australia (2018) List of specialties, fields of specialty practice and related specialist titles, www.medicalboard.gov.au/registration/types/specialist-registration/medical-specialties-and-specialty-fields.aspx

Melkas, H., Hennala, L., Pekkarinen, S. and Kyrki, V. (2020) Impacts of robot implementation on care personnel and clients in elderly-care institutions. *International Journal of Medical Informatics* 134: 104041. www.sciencedirect.com/science/article/pii/S1386505619300498

Menz, H., Borthwick, A. M., Potter, M. J., Landorf, K. B. and Munteanu, S. E. (2010) 'Foot' and 'surgeon': a tale of two definitions. *Journal of Foot and Ankle Research* 3(30).

Merrifield, N. (2018) 'Historic decision' by regulator to bring in raft of changes to nurse education, www.nursingtimes.net/news/education/historic-decision-by-nmc-brings-in-raft-of-nurse-education-changes/7023913.article

Millerson, G. (1964) *Qualifying Associations*, Oxon: Routledge.

Milligan, C. and Power, A. (2010) The changing geography of care. In: Brown, T., McLafferty, S. and Moon, G. (eds) *A Companion to Health and Medical Geography*, Oxford: Wiley-Blackwell.

Mitchell, D. (2019) A century of learning disability nursing. *Learning Disability Practice* 22(1): 11–13.

Montgomery, J. (2000) *Health Care Law*, Oxford: Oxford University Press.

Moore, H. R. (2018) Using holistic admission practices in radiologic technology programs to diversify the profession. PhD thesis, University of Cincinnati.

Moran, A. M., Nancarrow, S. A., Wiseman, L., Maher, K., Boyce, R. A., Borthwick, A. M. and Murphy, K. (2012) Assisting role redesign: a qualitative evaluation of the implementation of a podiatry assistant role to a community health setting utilising a traineeship approach. *Journal of Foot and Ankle Research* 5(1): 30.

Morrison, T. (1994) *Playing in the Dark: Whiteness and the Literary Imagination*, New York, NY: Vintage.

Mulligan, W. H. (1981) Mechanization and work in the American shoe industry: Lynn, Massachusetts, 1852–1883. *The Journal of Economic History* 41(1): 59–63.

Murphy, R. (1986) Weberian closure theory: a contribution to the ongoing assessment. *British Journal of Sociology* 37: 21–41.

Muzzin, L. J., Brown, G. P. and Hornosty, R. W. (1994) Consequences of feminization of a profession: the case of Canadian pharmacy. *Women & Health* 21(2/3): 39–56.

Nancarrow, S. (2004) Dynamic role boundaries in intermediate care services. *Journal of Interprofessional Care* 18(2): 141–51.

Nancarrow, S. (2015) Six principles to enhance health workforce flexibility. *Human Resources for Health* 13(1): 9.

Nancarrow, S. (2020) The interface of health support workers with the allied health professions. In: Saks, M. (ed) *Support Workers in the Healthcare Workforce: International Perspectives on the Invisible Providers of Healthcare*, Bristol: Policy Press.

Nancarrow, S. and Borthwick, A. M. (2005) Dynamic professional boundaries in the healthcare workforce. *Sociology of Health and Illness* 27(7): 897–919.

Nancarrow, S. and Mackey, H. (2005) The introduction and evaluation of an occupational therapy assistant practitioner. *Australian Occupational Therapy Journal* 52(4): 293–301.

Nancarrow, S., Moran, A., Wiseman, L., Pighills, A. C. and Murphy, K. (2012) Assessing the implementation process and outcomes of newly introduced assistant roles: a qualitative study to examine the utility of the Calderdale Framework as an appraisal tool. *Journal of Multidisciplinary Healthcare* 5: 307–17.

Nancarrow, S., Young, G., O'Callaghan, K., Jenkins, M., Philip, K. and Barlow, K. (2017) Shape of allied health: an environmental scan of 27 allied health professions in Victoria. *Australian Health Review* 41(3): 327–35.

National Alliance of Self Regulating Health Professions (2020) About NASRHP, https://nasrhp.org.au/about-us/

National Disability Scheme (2013) *Annual Report 2012–23*, Canberra: National Disability Scheme.

Navarro, V. (1978) *Class Struggle, the State and Medicine: An Historical and Contemporary Analysis of the Medical Sector in Great Britain*, London: Martin Robertson.

Navarro, V. (1986) *Crisis, Health, and Medicine: A Social Critique*, New York, NY: Tavistock.

Needle, J., Lawrenson, J. G. and Petchey, R. (2007) *Scope and Therapeutic Practice: A Survey of UK Optometrists: A Report Prepared for the College of Optometrists*, London: City of London University.

Nettleton, S. (1992) *Power, Pain and Dentistry*, Buckingham: Open University Press.

Nettleton, S. (1997) Governing the risky self. In: Petersen, A. and Bunton, R. (eds) *Foucault, Health and Medicine*, London: Routledge.

Nevile, A., Malbon, E., Kay, A. and Carey, G. (2019) The implementation of complex social policy: institutional layering and unintended consequences in the National Disability Insurance Scheme. *Australian Journal of Public Administration* 78(4): 562–76.

NHS England (2017) Chief Allied Health Professions Officer extends her remit to two additional professions, www.england.nhs.uk/2017/04/chief-allied-health-professions-officer-extends-her-remit-to-two-additional-professions/

Nicholls, D. A. (2018) *The End of Physiotherapy*, Abingdon: Routledge.

Nicholls, D. A. and Cheek, J. (2006) Physiotherapy and the shadow of prostitution: the Society of Trained Masseuses and the massage scandals of 1894. *Social Science & Medicine* 62(9): 2336–48.

Nicholls, D. A. and Gibson, B. E. (2010) The body and physiotherapy. *Physiotherapy Theory and Practice* 26(8): 497–509.

Nicholls, D. A. and Holmes, D. (2012) Discipline, desire, and transgression in physiotherapy practice. *Physiotherapy Theory and Practice* 28(6): 454–65.

Nicholson, S. L., Hayes, M. J. and Taylor, J. A. (2016) Cultural competency education in academic dental institutions in Australia and New Zealand: a survey study. *Journal of Dental Education* 80(8): 966–74.

Nielson, I. (2014) *Rural and Remote Generalist: Allied Health Project*, Cairns: Greater Northern Australia Regional Training Network. https://www.health.qld.gov.au/__data/assets/pdf_file/0025/656035/GNARTN-project-report.pdf

Noordegraaf, M. (2007) From 'pure' to 'hybrid' professionalism: present-day professionalism in ambiguous public domains. *Administration & Society* 39(6): 761–85.

Noordegraaf, M. (2016) Reconfiguring professional work: changing forms of professionalism in public services. *Administration & Society* 48(7): 783–810.

Numerato, D., Salvatore, D. and Fattore, G. (2012) The impact of management on medical professionalism: a review. *Sociology of Health and Illness* 34(4): 626–44.

Olgiati, V. (2010) The concept of profession today: a disquieting misnomer? *Comparative Sociology* 9: 804–42.

Olofsson, G. (2016) The expansion of the university sector, the emerging professions and the new professional landscape: the case of Sweden. PhD thesis, Department of Social Studies, Linnaeus University.

Olson, S. (2012) *Allied Health Workforce and Services: Workshop Summary*, Washington DC: National Academies Press. https://www.nap.edu/catalog/13261/allied-health-workforce-and-services-workshop-summary

Onyemaechi, N. O., Itanyi, I. U., Ossai, P. O. and Ezeanolue, E. E. (2020) Can traditional bonesetters become trained technicians? Feasibility study among a cohort of Nigerian traditional bonesetters. *Human Resources for Health* 18(1): 1–8.

Ottosson, A. (2016) One history or many herstories? Gender politics and the history of physiotherapy's origins in the nineteenth and early twentieth century. *Women's History Review* 25(2): 296–319.

Pain, T., Patterson, S., Kuipers, P. and Cornwell, P. (2018) Evaluation of the state-wide implementation of an allied health workforce redesign system: utilisation of the Calderdale Framework. *Asia Pacific Journal of Health Management* 13(3): 1.

Parker, J. M. and Hill, M. N. (2017) A review of advanced practice nursing in the United States, Canada, Australia and Hong Kong Special Administrative Region (SAR), China. *International Journal of Nursing Sciences* 4(2): 196–204.

Parkin, F. (1979) *Marxism and Class Theory: A Bourgeois Critique*, London: Tavistock.

Parkin, F. (1982) *Max Weber*, London: Routledge.

Parkin, F. (2002) *Max Weber* (rev edn), London and New York, NY: Routledge.

Parsons, T. (1991) *The Social System*, London: Routledge.

Payne, K. (1998) A pilot study of gender inequalities related to radiography education and career progression. *Radiography* 4(4): 279–87.

Peloquin, S. (1989) Sustaining the art of practice in occupational therapy. *American Journal of Occupational Therapy* 43(4): 219–26.

Peterson, J. B. (2018) *12 Rules for Life: An Antidote to Chaos*, London: Penguin Books.

Philip, K. (2015) Allied health: untapped potential in the Australian health system. *Australian Health Review* 39(3): 244–7.

Physiotherapy Board of New Zealand (2020) Specialisation, www.physioboard.org.nz/i-want-to-be-registered/specialist

Pickard, S. (2010) The role of governmentality in the establishment, maintenance and demise of professional jurisdictions: the case of geriatric medicine. *Sociology of Health & Illness* 32(7): 1072–86.

Pighills, A. C., Bradford, M., Bell, K., Flynn, L. J., Williams, G., Hornsby, D., Torgerson, D. J. and Kaltner, M. (2015) Skill-sharing between allied health professionals in a community setting: a randomised controlled trial. *International Journal of Therapy and Rehabilitation* 22(11): 524–34.

Pitama, S. G., Palmer, S. C., Huria, T., Lacey, C. and Wilkinson, T. (2018) Implementation and impact of indigenous health curricula: a systematic review. *Medical Education* 52(9): 898–909.

Porter, J. (2014) Transdisciplinary screening and intervention for nutrition, swallowing, cognition and communication: a case study. *Journal of Research in Interprofessional Practice and Education* 4(2), https://jripe.org/index.php/journal/article/view/152

Poulantzas, N. (1975) *Classes in Contemporary Capitalism*, London: New Left Books.

Price-Haywood, E. G., Burton, J., Fort, D. and Seoane, L. (2020) Hospitalization and mortality among black patients and white patients with COVID-19. *New England Journal of Medicine* 382: 2534–43.

Productivity Commission (2011) *Disability Care and Support*, Report no. 54, Canberra. https://www.pc.gov.au/inquiries/completed/disability-support/report/disability-support-volume1.pdf

Quilty, S., Valler, D. and Attia, J. (2014) Rural general physicians: improving access and reducing costs of health care in the bush. *Australian Health Review* 38(4): 420–4.

Rajan, P. (2014) Evolution of community physiotherapy in India. *Disability, CBR & Inclusive Development* 25(2): 97–104.

Randall, G. E. and Kindiak, D. H. (2008) Deprofessionalization or postprofessionalization? Reflections on the state of social work as a profession. *Social Work in Health Care* 47(4): 341–54.

Register, S. J. (2010) Optometric student gender trends and the importance of diversity: the impact of women in a male-dominated profession. *Optometric Education* 35(3): 108–11.

Riska, E. (2001) Towards gender balance: but will women physicians have an impact on medicine? *Social Science & Medicine* 52(2): 179–87.

Rogers, A. T., Bai, G., Lavin, R. A. and Anderson, G. F. (2017) Higher hospital spending on occupational therapy is associated with lower readmission rates. *Medical Care Research and Review* 74(6): 668–86.

Ross, K., Camara, K., Waldron, S. and Kime, N. (2016) The evolving role of the diabetes educator. *Diabetes Care for Children and Young People* 5: 23–8.

Royal College of Radiologists (2015) *Consultations on Proposals to Introduce Independent Prescribing by Radiographers across the United Kingdom: Response by the Royal College of Radiographers*, London: RCR.

Rumney, N. (2019) Optometry and independent prescribing. *Journal of Prescribing Practice* 1(2): 87–92.

Saks, M. (1983) Removing the blinkers? A critique of recent contributions to the sociology of the professions. *Sociological Review* 31(1): 1–21.

Saks, M. (1995) *Professions and the Public Interest: Medical Power, Altruism and Alternative Medicine*, London: Routledge.

Saks, M. (1999) The wheel turns? Professionalisation and alternative medicine in Britain. *Journal of Interprofessional Care* 13(2): 129–38.

Saks, M. (2003) The limitations of the Anglo–American sociology of the professions: a critique of the current neo-Weberian orthodoxy. *Knowledge, Work and Society* 1(1): 13–31.

Saks, M. (2010) Analyzing the professions: the case for the neo-Weberian approach. *Comparative Sociology* 9(6): 887–915.

Saks, M. (2012) Defining a profession: the role of knowledge and expertise. *Professions and Professionalism* 2: 1–10.

Saks, M. (2013) The limitations of the Anglo–American sociology of the professions: a critique of the current neo-Weberian orthodoxy. *Knowledge, Work and Society* 1(1): 13–31.

Saks, M. (2014) Regulating the English healthcare professions: zoos, circuses or safari parks? *Journal of Professions and Organization* 1(1): 84–98.

Saks, M. (2015) *The Professions, State and the Market*, Oxford: Routledge.

Saks, M. (2016) Professions and power: a review of theories of professions and power. In: Dent, M., Bourgeault, I., Denis, J. and Kuhlmann, E. (eds) *The Routledge Companion to the Professions and Professionalism*, Oxford: Routledge.

Saks, M. (2017) Slaying the Minotaur: reflections on the sociology of the professions. In: Liljegren, A. and Saks, M. (eds) *Professions and Metaphors: Understanding Professions in Society*, London: Routledge.

Saks, M. (2018) Regulation and Russian medicine: whither medical professionalism? In: Chamberlain, J.M., Dent, M. and Saks, M. (eds) *Professional Health Regulation in the Public Interest*, Bristol: Policy Press.

Saks, M. (2020) *Support Workers and the Health Professions: The Invisible Providers of Health Care*, Bristol: Policy Press.

Saks, M. and Allsop, J. (2007) Social policy, professional regulation and health support work in the United Kingdom. *Social Policy and Society* 6(2): 165–77.

Salvatore, D., Numerator, D. and Fattore, G. (2018) Physicians' professional autonomy and their organizational identification with their hospital. *BMC Health Services Research* 18(775).

Salvatori, P. (2001) The history of occupational therapy assistants in Canada: a comparison with the United States. *Canadian Journal of Occupational Therapy* 68(4): 217–27.

Savant, S. C., Hegde, S., Shirahatti, R. V. and Agarwal, D. (2016) Cultural competency amongst dental practitioners in Mumbai – a kap study. *Journal of Ahmedabad Dental College and Hospital* 7: 34–41.

Saxon, R. L., Gray, M. A. and Oprescu, F. I. (2014) Extended roles for allied health professionals: an updated systematic review of the evidence. *Journal of Multidisciplinary Healthcare* 7: 479.

Schofield, T. (2009) Gendered organizational dynamics: the elephant in the room for Australian allied health workforce policy and planning? *Journal of Sociology* 45(4): 383–400.

Shams-Avari, P. (2005) Linguistic and cultural competency. *Radiologic Technology* 76(6): 1–3.

Shield, F., Enderby, P. and Nancarrow, S. (2006) Stakeholder views of the training needs of an interprofessional practitioner who works with older people. *Nurse Education Today* 26(5): 367–76.

Short, S., Marcus, K. and Balasubramanian, M. (2016) Health workforce migration in the Asia Pacific: implications for the achievement of sustainable development goals. *Asia Pacific Journal of Health Management* 11(3): 58.

Shortell, S. M. (1974) Occupational prestige differences within the medical and allied health professions. *Social Science & Medicine (1967)* 8(1): 1–9.

Skills for Health (no date) Career framework, www.skillsforhealth.org. uk/careerframework/key_elements.php

Skinner, E. H., Haines, K. J., Hayes, K., Seller, D., Toohey, J. C., Reeve, J. C., Holdsworth, C. and Haines, T. P. (2015) Future of specialised roles in allied health practice: who is responsible? *Australian Health Review* 39(3): 255–9.

Smith, A. C., Thomas, E., Snoswell, C. L., Haydon, H., Mehrotra, A., Clemensen, J. and Caffery, L. J. (2020) Telehealth for global emergencies: implications for coronavirus disease 2019 (COVID-19). *Journal of Telemedicine and Telecare* 26(5): 309–13.

Smith, R. and Duffy, J. (2010) Developing a competent and flexible workforce using the Calderdale Framework. *International Journal of Therapy and Rehabilitation* 17(5): 254–62.

Smith, T. (2009) A short history of the origins of radiography in Australia. *Radiography* 15: e42–7.

Smith, T. and Baird, M. (2007) Radiographers' role in radiological reporting: a model to support future demand. *Medical Journal of Australia* 186(12): 629–31.

Smith, T., Fowler Davis, S., Nancarrow, S., Ariss, S. and Enderby, P. (2019) Towards a theoretical framework for integrated team leadership (IgTL). *Journal of Interprofessional Care*, DOI: 10.1080/13561820.2019.1676209

Snyder, M. M., Murphy-Nugen, A., Rose, A., Wells, G. and Mackusick, C. (2017) Implementation of competency based educational strategies into a first-year seminar for interprofessional healthcare science majors. *Internet Journal of Allied Health Sciences and Practice* 15(3): 4.

Sobo, E. J., Lambert, H. and Heath, C. D. (2020) More than a teachable moment: Black Lives Matter. *Anthropology & Medicine*: 27(3): 1–6.

Somerville, L., Davis, A., Milne, S., Terrill, D. and Philip, K. (2018) Exploration of an allied health workforce redesign model: quantifying the work of allied health assistants in a community workforce. *Australian Health Review* 42(4): 469–74.

Speech Pathology Australia (2001) Competency-based occupational standards (CBOS) for speech pathologists: entry level, Speech Pathology Australia.

Spink, M. J., Menz, H. B., Fotoohabadi, M. R., Wee, E., Landorf, K. B., Hill, K. D. and Lord, S. R. (2011) Effectiveness of a multifaceted podiatry intervention to prevent falls in community dwelling older people with disabling foot pain: randomised controlled trial. *BMJ* 342, DOI: https://doi.org/10.1136/bmj.d3411

Stapleford, J. and Todd, C. (1998) Why are there so few ethnic minority speech and language therapists? *International Journal of Language & Communication Disorders* 33(S1): 261–6.

State of Victoria Department of Health and Human Services (2016) Allied health: Credentialling, Competency and Capability Framework (revised edition): driving effective workforce practice in a changing health environment. Melbourne, Victoria.

Styhre, A. and Eriksson-Zetterquist, U. (2008) Thinking the multiple in gender and diversity studies: examining the concept of intersectionality. *Gender in Management: An International Journal* 23(8): 567–82.

Sudmann, T. T. (2009) (En)Gendering body politics. Physiotherapy as a window on health and illness. PhD thesis, University of Bergen.

Szreter, S. (1999) Rapid economic growth and 'the four Ds' of disruption, deprivation, disease and death: public health lessons from nineteenth-century Britain for twenty-first-century China? *Tropical Medicine & International Health* 4(2): 146–52.

Tawiah, A., Borthwick, A. and Woodhouse, L. (2020) Advanced physiotherapy practice: a qualitative study on the potential challenges and barriers to implementation in Ghana. *Physiotherapy Theory and Practice* 36(2): 307–15.

The Coalition of Health Professionals (2001) Mission statement of the Coalition of Health Professionals.

The Honourable Cordwainers' Company (2020) Home page, www.thehcc.org/framelss.htm

Thylefors, I., Persson, O. and Hellström, D. (2005) Team types, perceived efficiency and team climate in Swedish cross-professional teamwork. *Journal of Interprofessional Care* 19(2): 102–14.

Timmermans, S. and Berg, M. (2010) *The Gold Standard: The Challenge of Evidence-Based Medicine and Standardization in Health Care*, Philadelphia: Temple University Press.

Timmons, S. (2011) Professionalization and its discontents. *Health* 15(4): 337–52.

Timmons, S. and Tanner, J. (2004) A disputed occupational boundary: operating theatre and operating department practitioners. *Sociology of Health and Illness* 26(5): 645–66.

Timmons, S. and Tanner, J. (2008) Occupational boundaries in the operating theatre. *The Sociology of Healthcare: A Reader for Health Professionals* 277.

Titcomb, L. and Lawrenson, J. G. (2006) Recent changes in medicines legislation that affect optometrists. *Optometry in Practice* 7: 23–34.

Torstendahl, R. (1990) *The Formation of Professions: Knowledge, State and Strategy*, London: Sage.

Traynor, M. (2009) Indeterminacy and technicality revisited: how medicine and nursing have responded to the evidence-based movement. *Sociology of Health and Illness* 31(4): 494–507.

Truong, M. and Fuscaldo, G. (2012) Optometrists' perspectives on cross-cultural encounters in clinical practice: a pilot study. *Clinical and Experimental Optometry* 95(1): 37–42.

Truong, M. and Selig, S. (2017) Advancing cultural competence in optometry. *Clinical and Experimental Optometry* 100(4): 385–7.

Turner, B. (1985) Knowledge, skills and occupational strategy: the professionalisation of paramedical groups. *Community Health Studies* 9(1): 38–47.

Turner, B. (1995) *Medical Power and Social Knowledge*, London: Sage.

Turner, B. S. (1997) What is the sociology of the body. *Body and Society* 3(1): 103–7.

Turner, P. (2001) The occupational prestige of physiotherapy: perceptions of student physiotherapists in Australia. *Australian Journal of Physiotherapy* 47(3): 191–7.

Valentine, V., Kulkarni, K. and Hinnen, D. (2003) Evolving roles: from diabetes educators to advanced diabetes managers. *The Diabetes Educator* 29(4): 598–610.

Von Zweck, C. (1998) Support personnel in occupational therapy: who, what, why and how. *Canadian Journal of Occupational Therapy* 65(2): 59–63.

Wales, D., Skinner, L. and Hayman, M. (2017) The efficacy of telehealth-delivered speech and language intervention for primary school-age children: a systematic review. *International Journal of Telerehabilitation* 9(1): 55.

Watson, T. (1995) *Sociology, Work and Industry*, London: Routledge.

Webb, F., Farndon, L., Borthwick, A., Nancarrow, S. and Vernon, W. (2004) The development of support workers in allied health care: a case study of podiatry assistants. *British Journal of Podiatry* 7(3): 83–7.

Webster, C. (2002) *The National Health Service: A Political History*, Oxford: Oxford University Press.

Wiesel, I., Whitzman, C., Bigby, C. and Gleeson, B. (2017) *How Will the NDIS Change Australian Cities?*, Melbourne: Sustainable Society Institute.

Wilensky, H. L. (1964) The professionalization of everyone? *American Journal of Sociology* 70(2): 137–58.

Wilenski, P. (1976) *Delivery of Health Services in the People's Republic of China*, Ottawa, ON, CA: International Development Research Centre.

Willis, E. (1983) *Medical Dominance: The Division of Labour in Australian Healthcare*, Sydney: George Allen and Unwin.

Willis, E. (1989) *Medical Dominance: The Division of Labour in Australian Health Care* (2nd edn), Sydney: Allen & Unwin.

Willis, E. (2006) Introduction: taking stock of medical dominance. *Health Sociology Review* 15(5): 421–31.

Witz, A. (1992) *Professions and Patriarchy*, London: Routledge.

World Federation of Occupational Therapists (2012) About, www.wfot.org/about/about-occupational-therapy

World Health Organization (2013) *WHO Traditional Medicine Strategy 2014–2023*, Geneva: WHO.

Wright, A., Briscoe, K. and Lovett, R. (2019) A national profile of Aboriginal and Torres Strait Islander health workers, 2006–2016. *Australian and New Zealand Journal of Public Health* 43(1): 24–6.

Wyrley-Birch, B. (2006) The multilingual radiography classroom and the world of clinical practice. *Perspectives in Education* 24(3): 71–81.

Yamey, G. and Greenwood, R. (2004) Religious views of the 'medical' rehabilitation model: a pilot qualitative study. *Disability and Rehabilitation* 26(8): 455–62.

Yang, S., Shek, M. P., Tsunaka, M. and Lim, H. B. (2006) Cultural influences on occupational therapy practice in Singapore: a pilot study. *Occupational Therapy International* 13(3): 176–92.

Yeowell, G. (2010) What are the perceived needs of Pakistani women in the North West of England in relation to physiotherapy, and to what extent do they feel their needs are being met? *Physiotherapy* 96(3): 257–63.

Yeowell, G. (2013a) "Isn't it all whites?" Ethnic diversity and the physiotherapy profession. *Physiotherapy* 99(4): 341–6.

Yeowell, G. (2013b) "Oh my gosh I'm going to have to undress": potential barriers to greater ethnic diversity in the physiotherapy profession in the United Kingdom. *Physiotherapy* 99(4): 323–7.

Yielder, J. and Davis, M. (2007) Where radiographers fear to tread: resistance and apathy in radiographic practice. *Radiography* 15: 345–50.

Zagrodney, K. and Saks, M. (2017) Personal support workers in Canada: the new precariat? *Healthcare Policy/Politiques de Sante* 13(2): 31–9.

Zetka, J. R. (2003) *Surgeons and the Scope*, London: Cornell University Press.

Zetka, J. R. (2011) Establishing specialty jurisdictions in medicine: the case of American obstetrics and gynaecology. *Sociology of Health & Illness* 33(6): 837–52.

Zhou, K., Ma, Y. and Brogan, M. S. (2015) Dry needling versus acupuncture: the ongoing debate. *Acupuncture in Medicine* 33(6): 485–90.

Index

Printed and bound by CPI Group (UK) Ltd, Croydon, CR0 4YY

29/01/2025

14633483-0001